# COVID-19

## ADVANCE PRAISE FOR THE BOOK

'Clear, detailed, all-encompassing, elegantly written. Perhaps the most engagingly encyclopaedic compendium on SARS-CoV-2 in 260 pages' —Ambarish Satwik, author of *Perineum: Nether Parts of the Empire*

'A comprehensive scientific and sociological telling of one of the most disruptive events in our lifetimes. Anirban Mahapatra tells us how we got to this point, and where we go from here'—Sandeep Jauhar, author of *Heart: A History*

'In a world worn out by the pandemic and infodemic of COVID-19, Anirban's elegantly written book is a brilliant blend of science, history and sociological analysis that is rich in information and insights, while providing the pleasure of an easy read. It is strongly recommended for anyone who wishes to understand the dynamics of the present pandemic in the broader context of the human–microbial interactions that occurred in the past and may shape our future'—K. Srinath Reddy, president, Public Health Foundation of India

'*COVID-19: Separating Fact from Fiction* is an extraordinary book, both in content and composition. Anirban Mahapatra has analysed the vast body of scientific literature on COVID-19 that has accumulated in just less than a year and has written a definitive book on the most recent malady of our times. COVID-19 is unprecedented in the contemporary history of pandemics. We have seen fact meld into fiction, and this misinformation has impacted the basic fabric of human life. The talented author has brought together seemingly unconnected, complex aspects of the pandemic into a tightly woven book, in language that anyone can understand. The book cuts through news headlines and social media posts on COVID-19 to offer a calm and rational voice to the earth-shaking and unerasable human experience of the pandemic. This is a must-read for inquisitive minds across all ages'—Krishna N. Ganesh, professor of chemistry and director, Indian Institute of Science Education and Research, Tirupati

'This is a superb account of the origins, manifestations and lessons of the COVID-19 pandemic; it is deeply informative, highly accessible and engagingly written. Blending a meticulous understanding of microbiology, molecular biology and chemistry, Mahapatra guides us through the COVID-19 saga, offering vital lessons that we must embrace before the next pandemic strikes' —Kevin Davies, author of *Editing Humanity* and *The Sequence*

'Anirban Mahapatra's *COVID-19: Separating Fact from Fiction* is an engrossing narrative that integrates all the key scientific and societal aspects of the current COVID-19 pandemic with historical accounts of past viral outbreaks, and then relates these topics to the current state of affairs in India and the rest of the world. Accessible to all readers, Mahapatra walks [the reader] through all the basics of virology, vaccine development and divergent strategies to mitigate pandemics to create an essential guide for our times. Everyone should read this book to get a fuller understanding of living in a COVID-19 world'—Craig Lindsley, university professor of pharmacology, biochemistry and chemistry and director of the Warren Center for Neuroscience Drug Discovery, Vanderbilt University, Nashville, USA

# COVID-19

## SEPARATING FACT FROM FICTION

ANIRBAN MAHAPATRA

**PENGUIN**
**VIKING**

An imprint of Penguin Random House

VIKING

USA | Canada | UK | Ireland | Australia
New Zealand | India | South Africa | China

Viking is part of the Penguin Random House group of companies
whose addresses can be found at global.penguinrandomhouse.com

Published by Penguin Random House India Pvt. Ltd
7th Floor, Infinity Tower C, DLF Cyber City,
Gurgaon 122 002, Haryana, India

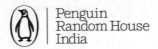

First published in Viking by Penguin Random House India 2021

10 9 8 7 6 5 4 3 2 1

While every effort has been made to verify the authenticity of the information
contained in this book, it is not intended as a substitute for medical consultation
with a physician. The publisher and the authors are in no way liable for the use
of the information contained in this book.

ISBN 9780670094370

Typeset in Adobe Caslon Pro by Manipal Technologies Limited, Manipal
Printed at Replika Press Pvt. Ltd, India

www.penguin.co.in

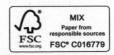

*For Arhan and Mitun*

# Contents

# 1

# Parable

'By hook or by crook this peril too shall be something that
we remember'

—Homer, *The Odyssey*

There is a well-known parable. A group of blind men approaches
an elephant. One feels the trunk and concludes that an elephant is
an animal like a snake. Another grasps one of its legs and discovers
that it is akin to a tree trunk. Yet another grabs an ear and describes
an elephant as a fan. A blind man grasping its tail thinks it is a kind
of rope. Touching the tusk, another remarks that an elephant is a
spear. The man who touches the side of an elephant is convinced
that an elephant is a wall.

A pandemic is an elephant described by nearly eight billion
blind people, each grasping at one or a few parts and trying to
make sense of the whole.

Some of us see in the pandemic signs of social reordering.
Others bemoan the moral decay that has occurred in people.
Some of us shake our heads in disbelief. Yet others need to pin
the blame on someone. Many of us see the Earth as a place that
would be better off without people. Some shrug it off with 'it's
not that bad. It will go away.' Others see it is as the end-of-times.

Our remembrance of this life-altering event—the likes of which the entire world has not witnessed in a century—what we think of it, how we feel about it and how we think we will get on once it is over is reflected by what we bring to the pandemic: our disposition, our experience, our background, and often, our privilege. Some of us were infected and fell sick. Some of us know someone who did not recover. Each of us will remember this pandemic differently.

The pandemic is biological, but it is also social. It is economic, but it is also political. Above all, we are facing a *human* pandemic, defined by both our collective humanity and inhumanity in the midst of an unexpected threat posed by a simple entity that follows evolutionary principles. Our world came to a grinding halt because of a virus that is exceedingly small. The virus has a compact genetic blueprint. The virus does not move on its own and needs to find new hosts. *The virus just needs to spread.*

In thousands of research articles in peer-reviewed journals and on scientific repositories that disseminate preliminary results, there are facets that are technical and medical. The print media highlights primarily socioeconomic dimensions. While following the pandemic on television and on social media, the angle is often political. When I read fictional stories or historical narratives, the voice is literary and introspective. And connecting all these threads in this current pandemic are our own fears for our relatives with medical conditions, and our aspirations for our children who look to us to answer why things are the way they are, and when they can play with friends and go back to school again.

From the start of the outbreak, we watched in horror as deaths mounted and as the threat mushroomed from country to country. By the end of 2020, SARS-CoV-2 had spread to over 190 countries. It had even reached Antarctica. Around 80 million cases had been identified. More than 1.7 million deaths had occurred. These numbers are of a magnitude that is difficult to comprehend.

In 2020, months felt like years, but one month stands out. In March 2020, the World Health Organization (WHO) declared that Severe Acute Respiratory Syndrome Coronavirus-2 (SARS-CoV-2), the novel coronavirus that causes Coronavirus Disease 2019 (COVID-19) had started a pandemic.[1]

During this chaos, I first approached the task of writing about the pandemic in the only way I knew how—by surveying the science of coronaviruses. This book is a snapshot of that knowledge. The picture may not be fully in focus, but it is no longer as blurry as it was on 31 December 2019, when the China office of the WHO was alerted of pneumonia of unknown cause that turned out be caused by SARS-CoV-2.[2]

Since then we have been living in extraordinary times when deciding to do simple things like going to a grocery store has become an exercise in real-time risk-assessment. And like everyone else there is the mental weight of decisions to be made—to take a flight, to visit an ageing parent, or to send a child to school.

Let me take you back to the early days of the pandemic. The defining symptoms of COVID-19 were initially thought to be mainly fever, cough and shortness of breath. At that time, public health officials had not advocated the universal wearing of facemasks in public. Transmission of SARS-CoV-2 had been reported to be less efficient than for influenza. The spread of the disease through aerosols was unknown, the effect of events where many people got infected at once had not been documented, and the disease was thought to be spread by those who were sick only after they got sick. India had not yet entered the largest lockdown in its history. In the United States, the ramifications of the initial failure to develop a diagnostic test that worked had not fully dawned on everyone. President Donald Trump and his family and colleagues had not been infected and had not recovered. The United Kingdom had not been gripped in fear over a new variant of the coronavirus.

In just one week in March 2020, global financial markets nosedived into bear territory, signalling a downturn. Economists revised their Gross Domestic Product (GDP) estimates downward. Cities and countries across the world closed borders to their own citizens, and to citizens of other nations. Gatherings were banned. The world stopped shaking hands. We worried about touching door handles and buttons on lifts. We stopped touching our own faces. World leaders recommended proper hand-washing techniques (the prime minister of the United Kingdom, Boris Johnson, who would later get infected and would recover, suggested singing 'Happy Birthday' twice to ensure that the ritual had been done for twenty seconds). Shoppers fought over the last few rolls of toilet paper in supermarkets in Western countries (and Indians observed this with a bit of curious bemusement). Meanwhile, India, the world's main supplier of generic drugs, restricted exports to store them up for its own citizens.[3] Hundreds of millions of children began missing school. We were entering a period of uncertainty in March, but the general sense on the street was that this would be over quickly.

From March through July, we learned more about COVID-19 and how it is unlike any other disease that we have faced before. We learned that symptoms also include loss of smell and taste, vomiting, diarrhoea, nausea and headaches.[4] We know much more about the trajectory of the disease and the spectrum of outcomes. We know that silent infections in those who never developed any symptoms of sickness and in those who will get sick later are a major way the virus is spread. Speaking of spread, in March, the consensus of public health officials was that the virus was spread by respiratory droplets expelled by coughing or sneezing, and from surfaces that had been infected with these droplets. By May, we had found out that we could not discount airborne spread, and that talking, singing and breathing expelled viruses.[5] By June, across the world, there was wider acceptance of facemasks as a preventative measure (with notable pockets of resistance in specific countries persisting). We also learned that as much as 80 per cent of those who are infected do not infect others: the virus is mainly spread by a few superspreaders and through 'superspreading' events.

The sheer number of scientific articles on COVID-19 that were published in 2020 is stunning. By mid-April 2020, the cumulative research output published on SARS-CoV-2 was doubling every two weeks.[6] On PubMed, the most popular database for medical research, there were more papers on coronaviruses in the first six months of 2020 than there had been in the preceding twenty years. By the end of the year, there were over 80,000 scientific articles and reviews on COVID-19, a disease that was unknown only a year earlier.[7] And even this is a skewed estimation of our recent interest in coronaviruses, because before the deadly outbreak of Severe Acute Respiratory Disease (SARS) in 2003, there were only a few hundred papers each year in the field. From being one of the 'backwaters' of virology, coronaviruses suddenly became something everyone at least knew something about.

But we can also marvel at the fact that faced with an unprecedented challenge, the world did seem to change overnight. Many people did rally to meet the challenges in a manner that would've been inconceivable even in January 2020. Many scientists I spoke to through the year from fields as disparate as materials science and chemical biology began to tackle scientific challenges posed by SARS-CoV-2. In the first major global health crisis of the social media era, epidemiologists were sought after online. Terms like 'social distancing' and 'flattening the curve' became part of the global lexicon. Almost immediately, many of us heeded the advice of public health experts to stay at home, wear facemasks and wash our hands. Businesses closed. Nonessential travel was discouraged. The world suddenly became insular.

As drugs and vaccines went into trials, different conventional approaches to control spread were employed, ranging from the early, strict lockdown in Wuhan, China, where infections were first observed to more laissez-faire policies—notably in Sweden, which allowed the virus to spread in the hope that immunity would be built up in the general population. At the end of 2020, life had returned to 'normal' in Wuhan.[8] Meanwhile, Sweden had admitted that its approach had failed to control infections and deaths.[9]

Around 150 countries imposed some form of a lockdown after the pandemic was first declared in March.[10] Most were eased by mid-June, often without fulling controlling transmissions. The epicentre of the pandemic shifted from China to Italy and then to the United States. Parts of Latin America, South Africa and Russia were hit hard. India reached a million confirmed infections in mid-July, and ten million before the end of the year.

Weeks of lockdowns turned into months. Hundreds of millions of jobs were lost. Amid it all, we realized that racial and ethnic minorities and the economically disadvantaged face a higher burden than others.[11] And in this time, we also saw the dark side of people who, even when faced with a health crisis, could not think beyond their immediate community or political inclinations.

Infections continued to rise globally. With over 5 million cases in European countries by mid-October, in a second surge that followed a summer slowdown, harsher measures were instituted. This second lockdown saw restaurants and bars closed, mandatory mask-wearing reinstituted where it had been relaxed, and restrictions on gatherings.[12] In mid-November, a week after the presidential election, daily reported cases topped 160,000 in the United States.[13] A study published that week pointed to restaurants, gyms and hotels as venues with the highest risk of spreading SARS-CoV-2.[14] By December, there was growing concern over a variant of the coronavirus that was spreading in the United Kingdom.[15] At the time of writing, it is thought that this variant is more infectious but there is no evidence that it causes more serious disease.[16]

Much is still unknown about the virus. Through most of 2020, there were conflicting accounts on whether infected children spread the virus as efficiently as adults (though a large-scale study in two states of India pointed out that there *can* be a high prevalence of infection in children).[17] The origin of the virus remained a subject of active inquiry. The robustness of immunity after infection was also being examined. We still did not have a handle on just how many people had been infected worldwide.

We have a better sense of the spectrum of COVID-19, but in 2020 we did not know why different people with no known risk factors suffered different fates. There were conflicting reports on whether the amount of virus that entered the body correlates with severity of COVID-19.[18] Scientists were also examining whether immunity conferred by infection from other common coronaviruses that circulate in people and cause colds offered some protection from SARS-CoV-2 infection.

There are also other mysteries. We know that those who are sixty years old and above, and those with chronic medical conditions, such as heart disease, diabetes and lung disease, have a higher chance of serious COVID-19. In an analysis of over a million reported cases, 14 per cent of people who were infected required hospitalization, so we know how many people get extremely sick.[19] But some young children and otherwise healthy people are also suffering and inexplicably dying. What are the genetic aspects that predispose certain people to more serious disease? Do they have aberrations in their immune responses? What makes them more susceptible than their peers? By the end of 2020, there were some breakthrough studies in each of these areas which are discussed in this book, but we have only scratched the surface.

We have also had a difficult time figuring out just how lethal COVID-19 is. The death rate varied dramatically over time and by region, estimated to be one out of ten reported cases in Wuhan at the start of the outbreak to one out of 2000 in Singapore from January to mid-July.[20] A whole host of factors determines outcomes, but there are no satisfying explanations yet as to why there is so much heterogeneity with infection. The good news is that physicians and caregivers got better at treating COVID-19, so the death rate fell towards the end of the year.[21] COVID-19 is no longer as fatal as it was when it appeared on the scene in Wuhan.

Still, simply looking at how many people die doesn't paint an accurate picture of COVID-19. One of the first studies out of China indicated that in around 80 per cent of patients, COVID-19 is an acute respiratory disease that clears after no or mild pneumonia. But later it became apparent that there are other long haulers, suffering from 'Long COVID' with debilitating symptoms months after the virus is cleared from their bodies. In addition, we know that COVID-19 is not just a respiratory disease. There is a wide variety of heart, blood, brain, skin, liver and kidney ailments that can occur. There is also variability in the immune response of cases, especially in the elderly. Details of why these occur is an area of ongoing, intense interest. But even in early 2021, *we just do not know.*

*How could this pandemic happen? How could we have missed the warning signs?*

You are not alone in wondering why we had not done more to stop this pandemic. There were certainly warning signs that had been ignored. At the turn of the century, coronaviruses were not thought of as a major threat. Much of the research funding in the West, at that time, went towards disease-causing organisms that could potentially be used as bioweapons such as anthrax or reengineered smallpox.

Much of that focus changed in 2002 with the SARS coronavirus epidemic which started in China and spread to two dozen other countries. In the end, 8,096 people were confirmed with SARS, and 774 died.[22] SARS spread quickly during specific events, air-travel and in hospital settings, seriously impacting healthcare professionals and the elderly. But with SARS, the world also got lucky. Because SARS was severe and spread mainly by people who were already sick, we did not have to worry about silent infections and it could be contained. In mid-2003, the epidemic was controlled, and no new cases have been observed since. Nevertheless, SARS was the first warning sign.

With new interest in coronaviruses, two human coronaviruses that cause mild common colds were identified. Suddenly, scientists began to look more closely at bats, thought to be the original source of SARS coronavirus. And then in 2012, yet another coronavirus emerged in people. The Middle Eastern Respiratory Syndrome (MERS) coronavirus, which started in Saudi Arabia, is transmitted from camels to people, but is also thought to have originated in bats.[23] MERS causes a severe disease but doesn't seem to spread very well in people. It is an ongoing outbreak with over 2400 infections and around 800 deaths so far.[24] MERS was another warning sign. But globally we were unprepared.

For over twenty-five years scientists and physicians had warned the public of a pandemic with many of the characteristics of COVID-19. In 2015, scientists and public health experts met in Geneva, Switzerland, to put together a list of emerging pathogens that might cause the next major outbreak.[25] The list included known viruses like Ebola, Nipah, SARS and MERS. In 2018, experts got together again to create the term 'Disease X' to describe a disease that might be caused by a new virus originating in animals. Disease X would be highly contagious and would result in more deaths among the infected than the seasonal flu. The experts did not know it then, but what they were describing was COVID-19. We are facing the first Disease X of the century.[26]

There are other well-documented proclamations spanning decades that experts can legitimately use to say, 'I told you so.' An article published in April 2020 pointed to twenty-five missed warning signs sounded by preeminent scientists, politicians and public figures through the years.[27]

Unfortunately, knowing that a pandemic might emerge is like predicting that hurricanes, earthquakes, tornadoes and terrorist attacks will occur. We can say reliably that they will happen. Knowing the specific details of when and where a new virus with the ability to cause a pandemic might originate is much harder to predict.

Just as we must document this experience, we must also learn from it. The pandemic has taught us about our place in nature. Most of us do not think about pandemics in normal times, but they do occur relatively frequently. In creating urban areas and through technological advances, we forget that we are part of the natural environment. And our own living conditions make us susceptible to infectious diseases, many of which cause pandemics.

Once SARS-CoV-2 began to spread well in people, we were at a disadvantage. While information and misinformation spread like lightning, the ability to control the spread of COVID-19 in the early months of the pandemic relied on much-slower tools— tracing of people who came in contact with those who were infected, isolation of patients and sanitation measures. These were the only effective tools in 2002–03, when I was a PhD student in microbiology and SARS became the first major infectious disease of the era of globalization. These were the same tools in 2009, when I wrote about H1N1 influenza, the first pandemic in my lifetime. They are all we had at the start of this pandemic. Unless we accelerate the search for pan-coronavirus and pan-influenza vaccines and drugs, these tools will be the only ones at our disposal when the next pandemic (possibly another acute respiratory infection caused by an RNA virus) strikes.

Still, I can't help but think about the scientific and medical response in the aftermath of the emergence of SARS-CoV-2. The genetic sequence of the virus was available in days. Vaccines went into clinical trials at a pace hitherto unseen in human history. We found out within months what tools the virus uses to get inside cells. We are learning valuable lessons on how to conduct drug trials. There were early missteps, but also successes. In a short span of time, we have found that there are drugs that work as treatments in specific cases of COVID-19; many others are in the process of being tested on people. Monoclonal antibody treatments have been approved after robust clinical trials.[28] We also must not forget that day after day, physicians and healthcare professionals have risked their lives to acquire this information and to treat the infirm.

But nowhere was the resolve more apparent than in the concerted and relentless effort in creating vaccines that would effectively offer protection to billions of people worldwide. From the moment the virus was known and its genetic material sequenced in early January 2020, scores of biotechnological and pharmaceutical companies partnered with academic scientists to create vaccines. Typically, vaccines take five to ten years to be commercially developed. Using different strategies, data from late-stage clinical trials involving tens of thousands of people started to come in quickly, and by November the first major vaccines had shown signs of success.[29] Vaccinations commenced apace in December.

We should step back and consider the dedication of these scientists. This is a remarkable feat without parallel in human history, since ultimately the production and deployment of safe and effective vaccines are key to ending the suffering caused by this virus.

What can we say after living with the virus for a year? There is much we already know. But a proper reckoning of the impact of COVID-19 on human health, society and the global economy will only be possible once viral spread has been controlled, and the pandemic has ended with the help of vaccines.

Bacteria and viruses will always infect us. COVID-19 is one of a long line of infectious diseases that have struck humanity. This is a sobering assessment and highlights the challenge that we face today. But COVID-19 is not the pandemic that will end civilization. It is not even the last pandemic that many of us will face.

But there will be light at the end of the tunnel. The pandemic is devastating, but it will end. My grandfather nearly died of typhoid when my father was young. My father lived through smallpox before I was born. Smallpox was eradicated by 1980, but not before killing more than 300 million people in the twentieth century alone. Typhoid is now treatable. Fighting infectious diseases is a never-ending battle that requires our sacrifices and our resourcefulness. So will fighting this one.

# 2

# Origins

It is difficult to come to terms with just how quickly COVID-19 irreversibly changed the world we live in. A good place to start a story is at the beginning. But where do you start when you do not know the beginning? We must start with the facts as they are known to us.

The first known cases of a deadly new pneumonia were associated with exposures in a live animal market in Wuhan, China.[1] Wuhan, with a population of 19 million, is the capital city of Hubei province, which has a population of 58 million. Most of these cases reported being ill with fever, though some had difficulty breathing. Chest imaging showed damage to the lungs in patients.[2] On 31 December 2019, as the world was preparing to usher in another new year, the WHO China Country Office was notified of multiple cases of pneumonia of unknown cause.[3]

The WHO believed at that time that there was no human-to-human spread, though that was later proven to be incorrect.[4] At that time, the virus that caused the pneumonia had not yet been identified or confirmed.

On 7 January 2020, a novel virus of the family *coronavirus* (first abbreviated as 2019-nCoV) was identified as the cause of the cases of pneumonia. Experts of the International Committee on Taxonomy of Viruses dubbed the 'novel coronavirus' SARS

Coronavirus-2 (SARS-CoV-2) based on genetic similarities with SARS coronavirus, which had arisen in East Asia and had wreaked havoc in 2002 and 2003.[5]

Just four days after the coronavirus was identified as the causative agent, the genetic sequence was officially released. This was an important milestone because having a sequence allowed a diagnostic test to be created to check for infections in people, the biological nature of the virus to be gleaned, and vaccines and drugs to be rapidly developed.

This was in stark contrast to the identification of the human immunodeficiency virus (HIV) which is the causative agent of acquired immunodeficiency syndrome (AIDS). The identification of HIV had taken years. Even years later, the identification of SARS took months. Because of the ease with which virus genomes can be sequenced, by September 2020 there were over 90,000 sequenced genomes of SARS-CoV-2 that scientists had examined to track mutations.[6]

Almost as soon as the causative agent of COVID-19 was identified in January, cases began to explode everywhere.[7] Although it was not known then, the virus had already spread and had been seeded globally, setting the stage for an unexpected global upheaval and an unprecedented counter-response. The death toll began to mount immediately. China responded swiftly by mobilizing doctors and nurses from across the country. By mid-January, most experts had come to terms with the potential for mass casualties. At that point, it was already known that COVID-19 was a serious disease with global implications.

On 23 January, Wuhan, the epicentre of the public health crisis, was put under lockdown. By the end of the month, as cases began to pop up in other countries, the world rose from its slumber. Travel to and from China was suspended. Unfortunately, by early January, SARS-CoV-2 had already spread to many parts of the world. Banning travel only limited new transmissions, akin to shutting the stable door after the horse has bolted.[8]

On 11 February 2020, the WHO announced that the disease caused by SARS-CoV-2 would be known as Coronavirus Disease 2019, or COVID-19. The WHO raised the threat from the coronavirus to 'very high' on 28 February, and declared a pandemic on 11 March.

There had been many warning signs. Scientists were aware of the significant potential of an emerging coronavirus to cause a pandemic. In the past few decades, two coronaviruses, those causing SARS and MERS, had jumped from animals to humans. But what exactly is it about coronaviruses that makes them likely to cause zoonoses—infectious diseases that can be transmitted from animals to humans?

Coronaviruses are especially promiscuous. These viruses have a propensity to infect multiple species of animals. There are four coronaviruses which cause many colds in people. However, repeated credible warnings by experts, and the experience with SARS, were ignored by policymakers.

So where did this coronavirus come from? To answer this question, scientists look at the genetic sequences of known viruses in different animals and see how they match up. If there is a strong match, it is possible that the two viruses are related. If there is a reasonably close match, we know for sure. So far there is no identified coronavirus in any animal with a perfect match to SARS-CoV-2 so we can't be absolutely sure.[9] But there are possible theories on its origin.

SARS-CoV-2 is about 96 per cent similar in terms of its genetic sequence to one kind of coronavirus found in horseshoe bats in Yunnan province in southern China.[10] So, it is quite possible that an early ancestor of SARS-CoV-2 might have originated there. Still, even though a 4 per cent difference in genetic sequence doesn't sound like a lot, based on the speed at which mutations accumulate and the size of their genomes, scientists have calculated that the bat coronavirus that they found in Yunnan and SARS-CoV-2 would've taken at least a few decades of evolution

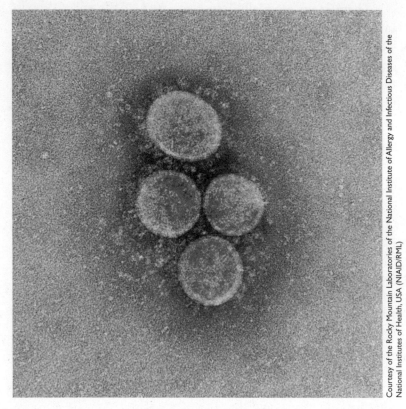

Courtesy of the Rocky Mountain Laboratories of the National Institute of Allergy and Infectious Diseases of the National Institutes of Health, USA (NIAID/RML)

Novel coronavirus, SARS-CoV-2

to diverge from one another. So, they are not the same virus. At best, they're related.

The fact of the matter is that simply looking at RNA sequences in coronavirus genomes is not enough. We also want to look at how these bases translate to amino acids in useful proteins. The success of the virus depends on its ability to infect cells, replicate and create new copies to repeat the cycle. The spike protein is responsible for the highly infectious nature of SARS-CoV-2 and it has a couple of features that make SARS-CoV-2 so successful. Comparing the amino acid sequences in different spike proteins is a way to deduce relatedness.

There is an especially important part of the spike protein, involved in recognizing a part of human cells that can be infected. This part of the spike protein is called the receptor-binding domain. No bat coronavirus that we have identified to date has the same sequences as the receptor-binding domain of the spike protein of SARS-CoV-2. So where did this sequence come from?

Yunnan province, where there are many horseshoe bats, is about 1500 kilometres from Wuhan, where the first cases were detected. So, there is a bit of distance between these two places. If SARS-CoV-2 ancestors did originate in Yunnan province, how on earth did they end up in Wuhan?

To answer this question, we can look at other coronaviruses that jumped from animals to humans in the last two decades. With the SARS coronavirus, a kind of animal known as a civet is thought to be the intermediate between bats and humans. Civets are sold in live animal markets in China where the disease originated in 2002. With MERS, camels acquired the coronaviruses (likely for decades) from bats. Could something similar have occurred with SARS-CoV-2?

It is certainly possible. The ecological and sequence separation of SARS-CoV-2 from known horseshoe bat viruses has led to two competing theories on its origin. One of these theories involves an intermediate species and the other doesn't.

In the first theory, a bat coronavirus infected an intermediate species before jumping to humans. Scientists think parts of the receptor-binding domain came from sequences of an animal other than a bat. And this is where it gets weirdly interesting.

Some scientists think a highly trafficked endangered scaly anteater called the pangolin is the intermediate species in the emergence of SARS-CoV-2.[11] A coronavirus found in pangolins has a near-perfect match for the very specific receptor-binding domain of SARS-CoV-2 spike protein. But overall, it only has a 90 per cent match for the whole virus.

So, in sum, SARS-CoV-2 appears to be mostly similar to a bat coronavirus genetic sequence, with an important sequence that it needs for infection similar to a sequence found in a pangolin coronavirus. How might SARS-CoV-2 have sequences that match two different coronaviruses in two different animals? Some scientists believe a bat coronavirus and a pangolin coronavirus infected one cell and the RNA genetic material recombined to form a hybrid virus. This SARS-CoV-2 ancestor may have taken the pangolin receptor-binding domain gene fragment and inserted it into the bat spike protein gene. This theory is plausible, but right now, it is also speculative because an intermediate has not been found.

The absence of a perfect match has prompted many to suggest that the virus was patched up in a laboratory from where it escaped. This is a controversial theory, but it cannot be formally ruled out until we find a match to SARS-CoV-2 in nature.[12] But we do not need to resort to this theory of deliberate genetic engineering, when a simpler natural one exists. Some viruses such as influenza viruses and coronaviruses mix and match different genetic pieces all the time. In fact, genetic mixing is what makes influenza subtypes acquire pandemic potential. Massive reassortment of coronaviruses in bats is known to occur too. Pandemics resulting from viruses that jump over from animals occur relatively frequently.

When did the virus first enter into circulation in people? Who was the first person to be infected? The early history of a virus that can spread stealthily among a susceptible population that does not yet know it exists is hard to reconstruct. Finding animals that contain coronaviruses that contain a high degree of genetic similarity, such as bats and pangolins, gives us a starting point to speculate. But it is quite possible that the virus may have spread in animals and people before mutations and chance encounters allowed it to cause the outbreaks detected in Wuhan in late 2019. Some scientists believe that the association is not straightforward and that before making a jump to humans, a predecessor of SARS-CoV-2 had been infecting another unidentified animal for decades.

This leads us to the second theory in which the origin of SARS-CoV-2 does not involve any intermediate animal.[13] According to this theory, both the pangolin coronavirus and SARS-CoV-2 came from the same ancestor. This theory postulates that SARS-CoV-2 is in fact a virus derived from bats that diverged from other known coronaviruses, anywhere between forty and seventy years ago. Over time, this ancestral coronavirus became SARS-CoV-2. Initially, people may have been exposed to the ancestral virus, but it would not have been very transmissible. More recent mutations may have sparked the changes that accelerated the pandemic.

Which of these theories is accurate? Until we identify every single coronavirus in horseshoe bats, we cannot rule out that the SARS-CoV-2 is uniquely a bat coronavirus. But if SARS-CoV-2 diverged from bats decades ago, we may not find an identical virus in those animals either. So, it is difficult to speculate currently.

But why are bats reservoirs of coronaviruses in the first place? Bats are one of the most prevalent mammalian species on the planet. Bats are also the only mammals with sustained flight. For reasons that are not known, bats tend to harbour a disproportionate number of viruses.[14] Many of the viruses that have jumped to humans have come from bats either by droplets, aerosols, faeces, or direct contact. The viruses that cause rabies, Nipah, Hendra and Ebola all came from bats.

There are different bat species across the world, and horseshoe bats have received much attention lately. Horseshoe bats are found in China and across Asia, and in many parts of Africa and Europe. Yunnan province is famous for the number and diversity of bats and the closeness of people with bats. It is estimated that there are over 5000 different bat coronaviruses, of which 500 are in China alone.[15] South-west China and South East Asia are the hotspots for the branching out of several new coronaviruses.

How can bats harbour so many different viruses? It is possible because these coronaviruses do not make bats sick. Why that is the case is a subject of ongoing investigation. It is currently thought that bats have special immune systems that help them cope with the stresses of flying that also keep them from getting serious coronavirus infections.

Being close to bats means people are exposed to bat viruses. Scientists can check for antibodies in people to see if they may have been exposed to coronaviruses. In a small study in a village in Yunnan, around 3 per cent of people had signatures of bat coronaviruses, suggesting that these coronaviruses may periodically jump to people.[16] Extrapolating from that small study to the total habitat of one kind of bat in Southeast Asia, it is possible to surmise that several million people have been exposed to bat coronaviruses. What this tells us is that in that part of the world, many people are often casually exposed to bats in a way that may make them more susceptible to being infected with bat coronaviruses.

Bats are rare in regular markets in China but are hunted and sold along with other exotic species in special live animal markets like the Huanan Seafood Market in Wuhan (which was frequented by some people who were infected in December 2019).[17] The market has since been disinfected and the animals there can't be sampled. Also, not all initially reported cases were tied to the market. We might need to go further back to identify the source of the first human infection.

We know that people can get infected by SARS-CoV-2. What about other animals? Currently, humans are the primary target of SARS-CoV-2. But by looking at genetic sequences of the virus, we can also make good guesses about which other animals might get infected by humans. Cats and ferrets have parts of cells, very similar to the ones in our cells, that the virus can use. So scientists predicted that they might also get infected.[18]

Quite remarkably, that prediction has held up. Cats and ferrets *do* get infected. In early April, four tigers and three lions tested positive for SARS-CoV-2 at the Bronx Zoo in New York.[19] It is quite likely that the seven animals were exposed to the virus from a zookeeper who was tending those animals. In December, three snow leopards tested positive in Kentucky.

There were also reports of two dogs that had been infected. Many scientists think infections in dogs are dead end events with no forward transmission to either other animals or people.[20]

There is a test for SARS-CoV-2 for dogs and cats that became available in mid-2020 in the United States. During the testing process, the two commercial laboratories that developed the test assessed thousands of samples without finding a single positive case.[21] All of this is good news for pet lovers.

What animals can be infected and serve as hosts also has implications for how we can control the spread of the disease. Smallpox was completely eradicated because only humans harboured the virus. We can imagine the same outcome eventually for polio. Even after vaccines for SARS-CoV-2 are administered to a large portion of the world's population, eradicating a disease becomes harder if the virus can hide in other animals and reinfect people intermittently. Right now, because of how well SARS-CoV-2 spreads in humans, we are infecting one another, but we should be concerned about animal reservoirs.

Minks are one such reservoir animal. A mink is a small ferret-like animal that is farmed for its skin. Minks can be asymptomatically infected with SARS-CoV-2.[22] Outbreaks in the Netherlands forced authorities to cull over 600,000 minks in June by suffocating them. The fear is that minks may cause a resurgence of disease in humans after the pandemic ends. A preliminary study in September 2020 indicated that minks had been infected by people, and then minks also infected some other people.[23] In November, Danish officials decided to kill millions of minks after reportedly discovering a mutation in animals infected with the virus.[24]

Another reservoir animal is the raccoon dog, which is also raised for its fur. There are over 14 million raccoon dogs in China. A study published in December determined that these animals are also susceptible to SARS-CoV-2 infection.[25]

All of this makes it unlikely that we might be able to eradicate SARS-CoV-2 completely.

# 3

# Coronavirus

Viruses are tiny entities which replicate. They are so simple that they do not possess the mechanism needed to do so, and so they must infect organisms which serve as hosts. All viruses are parasites by necessity.

The first virus detected was the tobacco mosaic virus in 1892. Back then, no one knew what a virus looked like. A virus was identified by physically passing an infected sample through a filter and discovering that what came out at the other end, the virus, was still infectious. Viruses were thus defined as being infectious agents that were too small to be trapped by a filter. The size criterion was used well into the early part of the twentieth century to classify viruses.

The first virus infecting humans to be identified was yellow fever virus back in 1900. Now we know that viral infections are relatively common. The technology for detecting viruses has improved by leaps and bounds since that time, so more and more viruses are detected each year.

Are viruses living? Well, that is up for debate. Viruses have no cellular structure. As you may recall from your school textbooks, cells are hallmarks of life. Viruses also have no known metabolism outside their hosts. Outside of hosts, they are inanimate nanoparticles. Viruses sit in a unique domain between simple molecules and living cells.

But within living organisms, they *act* like living organisms. Viruses reproduce, even though their form of reproduction is simply replication, a process by which copies are made of one parent virus. The rules of natural selection also apply to viruses in the same manner as they do to all forms of life. Viruses also have genetic material. All the information viruses need is in their genomes which contain either deoxyribonucleic acid (DNA) or ribonucleic acid (RNA).

DNA, which has two strands, is used by all living organisms as genetic material. Living organisms also have RNA, but RNA has mostly been relegated to other intermediate functions necessary for the creation of proteins, which are the building blocks and biological machines of life. Over the last few decades, we have also learned that RNA is also important in several different regulatory roles within cells.

There is no known form of modern cellular life that relies strictly on RNA as the primary genetic material. DNA is better suited for this role. The double-stranded nature of DNA allows for more complex organisms, such as humans, to exist. But there *are* viruses that use RNA. Some RNA viruses like influenza viruses which cause the flu have genetic material that is broken up into pieces. A few RNA viruses have two strands of RNA instead of one. Others like coronaviruses have one long RNA strand as their genetic material.

Typically, RNA viruses have very small genomes compared to other viruses, and this is one of the constraints of relying on RNA instead of DNA. RNA tends to impose a limit on the size of the genome, and by extension, on the complexity of the virus. RNA viruses are sloppy in how they replicate, giving rise to mutations. And because mutations can sometimes be harmful, their cumulative effects do not allow these viruses to expand their genetic material.

Because of the number of mistakes RNA viruses make during replication, they must make a huge number of copies of themselves to ensure that they are spread. Whether it is Ebola teeming in the blood of those who are infected, or influenza in a sneeze, RNA viruses tend to disperse in massive numbers.

Yet, even though RNA viruses are small and simple, they are not unsuccessful from a biological perspective. It is likely that *every* cellular organism, from bacteria to humans, from sponges to the largest trees on the planet, gets infected by RNA viruses.

Also, though RNA viruses are small, they utilize their genetic information very effectively. RNA viruses commonly have simple genomes with multiple proteins created from overlapping blueprint reading frames. As an analogy, you can think of a long sequence of bases in RNA as a long stretch of letters from which many overlapping words can be spelled out.

Where do RNA viruses come from? Viruses are thought to be modern holdovers from an ancient era, a so-called 'RNA World', which predates all living organisms. It is believed that roughly four billion years ago, RNA did the job that DNA does today in cells, but later, in more advanced organisms, it got relegated to roles it has in modern cellular life. The genetic role of the RNA World is retained in RNA viruses.

There is another more recent theory for the origin of certain viruses. The discovery of large DNA viruses such as Mimivirus and Pandoravirus that almost resemble cells also gives credence to the idea that some viruses might have come from stripped-down cells.[1]

All said, I hesitate to use the word 'primitive' to describe viruses. Though a virus may be simple, it is very successful in achieving its goal of spreading. Viruses are diverse and can readily adapt. In fact, viruses may even be considered the most successful types of biological entities.[2] Even in the human body, there are probably one hundred times as many viruses as there are human cells.

Now, a word about how RNA viruses replicate. Enzymes are protein machines that speed up chemical reactions, making all life possible. Different organisms use a swathe of different enzymes. Some enzymes are copiers that catalyse replication of genetic material. Because RNA viruses contain RNA as their genetic material, they cannot use enzymes which act as copiers for DNA genetic material inside host cells.

RNA viruses can get inside our cells, steal our resources and hijack our biological machines, but they need their own RNA copier—an enzyme known as RNA-dependent RNA-polymerase. This is a key actor in the life cycle of SARS-CoV-2 as well. (Most RNA viruses that infect people such as Ebola, influenza and SARS use this copier enzyme, but there are exceptions which convert their RNA to DNA first, such as HIV which causes AIDS.)

This enzyme is an attractive target for antiviral drugs. The idea is that if we can stop an RNA virus from making functional copies of its genetic material by hindering its copier enzyme, we have a shot at stopping the virus from replicating. Such a drug would be specific for viruses and not for our cells causing, in theory, few side effects. This is in fact the principle behind remdesivir (a drug created to treat Ebola) which is an antiviral drug that has been used for the treatment of SARS-CoV-2 infections.[3]

The polymerase RNA copier enzyme also makes a lot of errors, and so many of the bases get wrongly put in subsequent copies. These are mutations that can have implications for infection and disease. Mutation rates in RNA viruses are high. Humans and chimpanzees have a difference of about 2 per cent in genomic sequences that can come about after around 8 million years of divergent evolution.[4] An RNA virus without proofreading ability like polio virus can manage a 2 per cent change in its genetic material in just five days!

I mentioned that RNA viruses have small genomes. In biology, there are also often exceptions to rules, and a notable exception to the size limit of genomes for RNA viruses are a spherical type of viruses known as coronaviruses. Coronaviruses include SARS-CoV-2, which has a genetic script that is just under 30,000 bases, large for an RNA virus.

To make sure that fewer errors are made across the stretch of their relatively large genome, coronaviruses harbour the gene for a proofreading enzyme. This is not found in RNA viruses with genetic material less than 20,000 bases. Think of it as an autocorrect feature for the polymerase copier, and it is the reason that coronaviruses have a lower mutation rate than influenza viruses.[5]

A larger genome in coronaviruses also means that it has more genes than it might have had had it been smaller. More genes typically correspond with more proteins. Some of these coronavirus proteins (mostly enzymes) are part of the viral toolkit that makes it such an indefatigable foe.

SARS-CoV-2 was initially thought to have genes that give rise to twenty-nine proteins.[6] A scan of the genome in September 2020 turned up twenty-three more genes, many of which give rise to unknown proteins.[7] For some of the proteins for which we do not know the function, we can predict that they help the virus to trick the host immune system. Recent work has helped us to find out which human proteins SARS-CoV-2 proteins interact with, and this is an avenue of exciting, ongoing investigation in the identification of drugs.

By now, everyone knows that SARS-CoV-2 is a coronavirus. But what *is* a coronavirus?

Coronaviruses are spherical viruses that are about 60-140 nanometres in diameter. They are neither the smallest nor the biggest viruses. For scale, there are 1000 nanometres in one micrometre, and 1 million nanometres in one millimetre. The spike, which is shaped like a club, is the most prominent distinguishing feature coming out from the surface of the virus. Spikes make the virus look like the corona of the Sun.

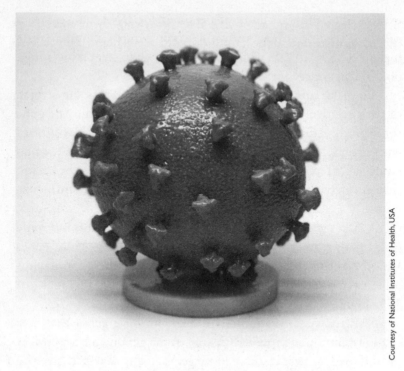

Courtesy of National Institutes of Health, USA

A model of SARS-CoV-2 with prominent spikes visible

The first coronavirus to be discovered was the infectious bronchitis virus. Identified in 1937, it is a virus which infects chickens. For decades, coronaviruses had been known to infect several animals, such as cows, pigs, dogs, cats and chickens, but not humans. That changed in the early 1960s when the first human coronaviruses were discovered. In people, coronaviruses mainly cause respiratory diseases, but in animals they have a host of symptoms causing respiratory diseases as well as gastrointestinal diseases such as haemorrhagic diarrhoea.

The discovery of the first human coronavirus is an intriguing story. British virologist David Tyrrell had been studying the common cold at a facility in Salisbury, UK, called the Common Cold Unit (CCU).[8] From 1946 to 1990, over 20,000 volunteers were selected to spend a few days in a trial where tests on the transmission of the common cold were being conducted. Some were purposely infected with viruses that cause the common cold.

While researching the common cold, scientists at the CCU made the astonishing discovery that it is not caused by one virus, but by *hundreds* of them, virtually quashing hopes of a vaccine, because a vaccine is often created specifically for one invader. Working at the CCU, Tyrrell, along with colleague Malcolm Bynoe, isolated a virus from the nasal swab of a boy. The virus was seen for the first time by June Almeida (née Hart), a brilliant virologist known for developing new methods for imaging viruses.[9] Together, with other scientists, Almeida and Tyrrell named the new family of viruses with the solar-corona-shaped spike, 'coronavirus'.

After that discovery, coronaviruses were mostly ignored. For decades, two coronaviruses named OC43 and 229E were the only two known to infect people. They cause a mild, self-limiting respiratory infection. Together, these two viruses are responsible for perhaps 10 per cent of the common colds and are likely to never be eradicated. Infections caused by these viruses are also seasonal: all of us know that we are more likely to catch a cold in the winter than in the summer. Since cold infections are typically mild and get better on their own, no one put in any significant effort in creating vaccines against human coronaviruses because the benefit simply would not justify the time and cost.

Everyone catches a cold. It is one of those ubiquitous infections. Children under the age of six catch around six colds a year; adults perhaps only half as many, having built up some immunity to many strains and being more hygienic in practices. More than 90 per cent of us have detectable antibodies to human coronaviruses OC43 and 229E, indicating that we have been infected with these coronaviruses perhaps multiple times in our lives. Infection does not confer lifelong sterilizing immunity, which means catching a cold from OC43 does not mean that you will not catch another caused by the same virus six months later.

Coronaviruses cause severe, fatal diseases in animals, and vaccines that protect animals against infections by various coronaviruses have been developed, so it's incorrect to think that there were no coronavirus vaccines prior to the SARS-CoV-2 pandemic. But by and large, coronaviruses were not the focus of intense medical inquiry. A story in *Science* even called coronavirology one of the 'backwaters' of virology.[10]

Then in March 2003, WHO issued its first global alert in ten years because a mysterious *atypical pneumonia* was killing hundreds of people in mainland China, Hong Kong and Vietnam. Atypical pneumonia is a blanket designation. The signs and symptoms of pneumonia can be spotted by a doctor in a clinic, and when there are many cases that do not have a known cause, they raise an alarm. Sometimes, these cases of pneumonia are due to a virus. COVID-19 also began as an abnormal number of cases of atypical pneumonia.

SARS-laden samples were taken from sick patients and the causative virus was cultured in laboratories by infecting mammalian cells. Using the high resolution of a technique called electron microscopy, scientists noticed sunlike spikes. These were the tell-tale signs of the coronavirus June Almeida identified many years earlier. Using genetic technologies, scientists confirmed that the infectious agent was a new virus belonging to the coronavirus family. Patients who recovered had antibodies that reacted with wide-ranging coronavirus antibody-generating parts, another confirmatory piece of evidence. The world had its first deadly coronavirus.

After SARS was identified, the next step was sequencing its genome. Back in 2003, next-generation sequencing platforms had not advanced to the current level of sophistication, so sequencing the viral genome was not straightforward.

There was no vaccine or drug for the SARS coronavirus, and it caused a profoundly serious illness resulting in many deaths. Within days of SARS spreading from mainland China to Hong Kong in February, international air travellers seeded outbreaks in Vietnam, Singapore, Toronto in Canada, and elsewhere. Ultimately, it spread to countries on five continents. Yet, as quickly as it arrived, by July 2003, the epidemic was over.

SARS was stopped because the virus wasn't a perfect adversary. It was infectious mostly after people got sick so isolating the sick and tracing contacts were enough to control it. It was deadly in the elderly with more than half of those above sixty-five years of age dying. Transmission within healthcare settings was a notable feature, accounting for 21 per cent of all cases. In children it was mild, similar to SARS-CoV-2 infection. No child died of SARS in 2002 or 2003.

SARS put coronaviruses on the map. The world finally understood the potential for new disease-causing coronaviruses. Where had SARS come from? Bats became known as a reservoir of these viruses. We learned that bat coronaviruses tend to jump to other animals, especially when live animals are near one another and near humans, such as in wet markets.

It is thought that SARS coronavirus spread from bats to civets, and then from civets to people. Few had bothered to look at bat coronaviruses closely until the emergence of SARS, but in the years since, bats have gained notoriety as a natural reservoir for coronaviruses.

Immediately in the aftermath of SARS, two other human coronaviruses, HKU1 and NL63, were identified. They weren't new viruses, but because no one had searched for them, they had not been found earlier. Like OC43 and 229E, these two viruses are responsible for seasonal colds and most people have antibodies to them.

Then in 2012, yet another coronavirus emerged in people. This time it was MERS in Saudi Arabia. Fortunately, this disease doesn't spread very well from person to person after emergence. Otherwise, there would be serious cause for concern. MERS is the most lethal coronavirus disease known to infect humans and has an estimated 35 per cent fatality rate.

More research on coronaviruses, particularly with respect to cures and vaccines, was warranted, including the development of all-purpose options that worked against a broad swathe of RNA viruses. Unfortunately, once the SARS epidemic was over, we moved on. The pharmaceutical industry is hesitant to fund research for diseases that do not exist yet, and governments want direct and immediate applications for research that they fund. It is this lack of foresight of our species that gets us in trouble time and again.

To recap, we knew about two coronaviruses which cause infectious diseases in humans back in 2002. The number of coronaviruses that infect humans grew to six by 2012. Going simply by the trend of emerging coronaviruses like SARS and MERS, we should have anticipated the emergence of other coronaviruses like SARS-CoV-2.

Scientists who study coronaviruses had warned us. In a review in 2015, two scientists, Anthony Fehr and Stanley Perlman, cautioned that coronaviruses would continue to emerge and cause outbreaks because of their ability to mutate, mix-and-match between strains and jump to different animals.[11]

Fehr and Perlman were not the only ones. In scientific articles published in 2015 and 2016, Vineet Menachery, Ralph Baric and colleagues discovered coronaviruses in bats that could jump to humans.[12] Although these coronaviruses are not directly connected to SARS-CoV-2, we should have anticipated the emergence of another coronavirus based on the accumulating mountain of evidence.

# 4

# Concepts

## Structure and function are related

This is going to be a very breezy introduction to a few concepts that we should know before we dive into a discussion of SARS-CoV-2 infection, human immunity, drugs and vaccines.

There is much that we don't know about the bewildering number of lifeforms on the planet both living and extinct. But all known life on earth follows certain rules and uses specific building blocks. Large organic molecules such as nucleic acids, proteins, carbohydrates and lipids are the stars of the show. Nevertheless, at a very fundamental level, life can be explained in physical and chemical terms through energy, matter and interactions. All these rules apply as much for SARS-CoV-2 as they do for us.

SARS-CoV-2 is not an alien lifeform from another planet with properties that make it difficult to identify. It obeys the same physical principles and uses the same broad classes of the large molecules we do. That is why the virus can recognize our cells and infect us, and in response, our immune system is usually prepared to tackle it.

One of the central themes of biology, at the level of molecules and atoms, is that structure is related to function. How a large molecule or a biological machine is shaped determines what it does and how well it does its job. If its shape is distorted it might not function well at all. And structures that do a job well are maintained across generations and different species.

The noted astrophysicist Carl Sagan once said, 'If you wish to make an apple pie from scratch, you must first invent the universe.' We can create a pie because matter and the fundamental laws of physics exist. If this framework did not exist, that would have to be created first. Instead of creating, for example, a completely new large molecule for a new job, an organism will find one in its toolkit that can be modified through the awesome power of natural selection.

Now, shapes are not the only aspect of course, there are other different chemical and physical interactions that go on, but for the sake of our discussion we will keep things simple and focus only on shape. How structure relates to function is an extremely complex three-dimensional puzzle. It is important to remember, however, that these structures are not rigid; they're moving dynamically and undergoing what are called conformational changes in shape.

*Enzymes* are a subset of proteins in all living organisms that speed up reactions. They make things happen. And for a century now, hundreds of thousands of biologists, pharmacologists and chemists have spent their professional careers studying these types of molecules and tying structure with function.

Specific shapes bring different biological molecules together. They also bring drugs into the active sites of enzymes where things happen. Many drugs work by tampering with the activity of enzymes. This too is related to the shape of the drug and the enzyme. Closely tied to shape are chemical interactions weaker than strong bonds (called non-covalent interactions).

Scientists talk about the genetic code in the form of four different letters or bases. And the genetic code gives rise to an intermediate molecule, RNA, which is usually translated by 'words' of three letters into twenty amino acids. Amino acids make up proteins. This might make it sound like proteins are written flat like paper, but they are layered and three-dimensional: more like origami. And this is brilliant because changes to the simple letters affect the three-dimensional structure and how a protein works. The ability to create such amazing complexity from relative simplicity is one of the most beautiful ideas on the planet and should also serve as a source of wonder and appreciation. It should be a rallying call for conservation.

How does all this relate to SARS-CoV-2? If the shape of a part of the virus (for example, the spike protein) has a decent fit with the shape of a part of the cell that will let it in (the cellular receptor), the virus can cause infection. If, on the other hand, the shape of a drug or antibody fits that same part of the virus better, it can stop the virus. This is a simplistic explanation, but a good way to grasp how drugs, enzymes and immunity work in biology at the level of atoms and molecules.

Let me give you one more example that is relevant to the current pandemic. *Antibodies* are protein molecules that latch on to parts of foreign invaders (*antigens*). Antibodies that attach to and prevent a virus from infecting cells are called *neutralizing antibodies* and protect people from reinfection with the same virus. Antibodies also have another job. They mark the invaders for destruction by cells of the immune system. Antibodies interact with antigens on virus surfaces mainly through small areas which have complementary shape and they can be extremely specific for antigens.

To stop SARS-CoV-2 from infecting cells, antibodies will recognize the shape of a part of the spike of the virus. But the virus will also evade them by decorating the spike with sugars that make it harder to recognize and access.

As a virus mutates, its important proteins change shape a little bit, trying to work better, but also to evade immunity. Because the interactions are so fine-tuned even small changes due to mutations can lead to a change in shape and to weaker binding by antibodies and lower immunity. A small change caused by a mutation can also result in more infectivity. Some mutations can cause vaccines to be less effective.

You may have wondered how the pieces of SARS-CoV-2 were deciphered. First, the virus was isolated from sick patients and identified visually. Then, it was taken apart and its genetic information was characterized. That simple code of letters was a treasure trove, because scientists could use it to simulate the shapes of its key enzymes. They used the information to get each of the genes of the virus and build up its architecture from the simple blueprint. They were also able to compare it with existing viruses. Simultaneously, they used it to extract the enzymes of the virus in genetically engineered hosts. They then painstakingly resolved the 3D structures of these key actors. With the shapes in hand, they are designing drugs by seeing how well synthetic chemical molecules fit in the business end of enzymes and modify their roles.

The relationship between structure and function is such an obvious and elegant unifying concept that it should be in school biology books. Except it isn't. I wish someone had told me when I was up at night memorizing minutiae for exams in school. In biology size does matter. And so does shape.

## Natural selection drives life

Having introduced the relationship between structure and function, I want to introduce another foundational concept that will help us to understand life through the lens of a biologist. Armed with this concept, you too will be able to think like a biologist.

The biological driving force of all life is evolution by natural selection. We like to think of evolution as a big change, for example, when one animal evolves into another, but the truth is it is happening all the time, and typically in small ways through mutations.

When mistakes happen to genetic material, they are known as mutations. They can be the result of copying errors or from mutagens. Unlike in films, mutations are usually boring: they don't bestow any superpowers.

Usually, in a population, whether it is made up of cells or viruses, there are a whole lot of mutations that do not make much difference. There are some that cause enough harm to kill, and those do not get passed on. For natural selection to act on a biological entity, it must be able to pass on copies of itself. Occasionally, there will be some that confer some advantage and those are the mutants that are most likely to live. As circumstances *always* change, some of the mutations in a population that didn't previously make a difference are going to give the organisms a selective advantage and get propagated.

This is a fundamental concept to understanding life. Elucidating it is one of the greatest intellectual achievements in history. Humans are products of evolution, and we discovered the process by which all other life evolved on this planet. I am convinced that if we discover life elsewhere in the universe, it too will bear the hallmark of being able to evolve though natural selection. As Theodosius Dobzhansky famously wrote, 'Nothing in biology makes sense except in the light of evolution.' We exist and thrive because of evolution, and sometimes when some of our cells become *too* successful we develop certain diseases such as cancers.

How does all of this relate to a virus like SARS-CoV-2? A virus is a tiny entity with an exceedingly small genetic component: it has a minimalist lifestyle. It doesn't really do much except infecting cells to get them to make copies of it. Any mutation that interferes with necessary pieces in its lifecycle is not going to be well tolerated. On the other hand, any mutation that lets it infect better gives it a boost and will likely be maintained.

Let us take a specific example relating to SARS-CoV-2. The spike is like a key that unlocks the door of cells to let the virus get inside. It is particularly important for the virus to be able to infect cells because if it can't, it won't be able to propagate. The spike is made up of three equal spike proteins. A mutation in the part of the spike protein that doesn't let it latch on to cells as easily is going to make it less infectious, and from the perspective of the virus, is unwanted. Conversely, mutations to the spike protein that help a virus infect cells better might be maintained.

The point to reiterate is that mutations are common in the genetic material of RNA viruses like SARS-CoV-2. What is reassuring from a human perspective is that mutations that might actually cause the creation of a new strain with enhanced spread or more severe disease are much less common.

One mutation in the spike protein, called D614G, emerged early during the pandemic, and became prevalent worldwide. It is an example where a change of a single amino acid in the spike protein of the virus resulted in a new mutant, G614. By the end of 2020, G614 became the dominant version of the virus in the world. Some experiments have demonstrated that this mutation facilitates the spread of the virus by making it easier for the virus to enter cells. In other words, this is a mutation that is beneficial to the virus and has been maintained in its genetic sequence.[1] This is plausible. That said, this variant is probably just as susceptible to vaccine-induced immunity as the strain that originated in China, so we need not worry about the effects on vaccines right now. Additionally, by the end of 2020, there was no sign that G614 causes more severe disease, but this warrants further investigation.[2]

In late 2020, another variant, which caused great alarm, was detected in the United Kingdom.[3] This variant has seventeen mutations in total and is believed to be more transmissible in people than other previously characterized variants of SARS-CoV-2. It is thought that this variant, which has many mutations that lead to a different spike protein, emerged in a single patient with a long bout of COVID-19. The detection of this strain led to harsher lockdown measures and restrictions on travel from the UK in December. At the end of 2020, researchers were frantically trying to determine if the new variant did, in fact, spread faster or cause more severe COVID-19.

# 5

# Emergence

Viruses of wild and domestic animals can infect humans by a process called zoonosis. While humans are constantly exposed to animal viruses, those that can successfully infect and transmit between humans are rather rare. Even when a virus enters a person, it must be able to spread. A short course of infection with high fatality and low spread would be limiting because the virus wouldn't be able to spread to the next person.

Much of the emergence of a disease is also a matter of chance encounters that bring a virus out of obscurity by selective advantage or proximity to new hosts. There are many viruses in the wild that could possibly infect people, but people must get exposed to them to be able to get infected.

Nearly all pandemics originate from a single source.[1] For infectious diseases that spill over from animals, one person or a few people must come in contact with an animal harbouring the disease-causing organism.

For a cross-species transmission to occur, a virus has to get past host immunity, infect a cell that it recognizes, create many copies of itself using the host machinery, exit the cell and find a way to spread to other people in the population. That last step relies on people behaving in certain ways.

RNA viruses are presently the most common cause of emerging diseases in humans. The ability to jump from one animal host to another is exceptional in RNA viruses because they mutate fast and make themselves at home in their new hosts. Transmission of different RNA viruses can occur through aerosols, bodily fluids like blood from slaughter of animals, insect vectors, or faeces.

Infectious diseases have always plagued humans. Our genetic material is dotted with the genetic archaeology of past infections. Approximately 8 per cent of our genomes comprise sequences that are viral in origin. It may come as a surprise to many people that genetically we're part virus ourselves.[2]

Parasites infected hunter-gatherer societies, but certain events in human history have certainly hastened the emergence and spread of infectious diseases in more modern societies.

Infections from RNA viruses must have been a major obstruction to human survival for our ancestors. Everywhere they went, they would've come in contact with new animals that spread viruses for which they wouldn't have had any immunity. And yet, through these pestilences, our ancestors persisted.

A major milestone in human history was the initiation of farming around 10,000 years ago. This breakthrough increased the number of humans that could be sustained on a parcel of land, paving the way for the crowded human societies we live in today. Farming of animals also put humans in sustained, close contact with domesticated animal species.

A second milestone in human history was urbanization, roughly 5000 years ago. Urbanization increased networks among possible hosts of viruses and provided conducive conditions for rapid spread of diseases. Most infections caused by RNA viruses are acute. Think of the flu or the common cold which are caused by RNA viruses. They tend to burn out quickly. Dense settlements would have been a major turning point for RNA viruses, facilitating human-to-human transmission during a short course of infection. A disease like measles, for example, wouldn't have become established in people without cities.

A third more recent milestone has been global travel. Travel and migrations facilitated both the emergence and establishment of infectious diseases. Plague first emerged in humans over 5000 years ago. The first major outbreak was during the time of the Roman Emperor Justinian in Constantinople around AD 541. It arrived with infected rats from Egypt on grain ships. Trade with Asia, through the Silk Route and in shipping routes, brought rats with bacteria causing the bubonic plague responsible for the Black Death. The Black Death started in Europe in the fourteenth century and is estimated to have killed more than fifty million people.

Tuberculosis (TB), which is the leading cause of death due to an infectious disease in people, was thought to have been caused by a bacterium whose predecessor infected our modern human ancestors before they left Africa 70,000 years ago. Cows are infected with various TB strains and can pass the disease on to humans. Whether cows first gave humans TB or whether our ancestors gave the germs to cows has been a source of much interest. More recent work indicates that TB may have emerged in humans from seals, and this possibly happened much later when people lived in close communities (in what is now Peru).[3]

Smallpox, which has probably only been circulating in humans for less than 4000 years, also spread through travel. It found susceptible populations among Native Americans, decimating entire habitations. It arrived in the Americas with European travellers. Slave trade brought the yellow fever virus from Africa to the Americas.

There are more recent examples as well. Zika virus is an RNA virus transmitted by a kind of mosquito. Prior to 2007, it had only been found in fourteen people, all of whom had mild symptoms. In 2015, Brazil experienced an unprecedented outbreak caused by Zika virus linked to travel originating outside South America.[4]

The occurrence of a specific birth defect associated with Zika infection, babies born with small heads, received widespread coverage. There were potentially over 1 million cases of Zika between 2015 and 2018. Airline travel probably seeded Zika in South America early during the outbreak.

Crowded spaces also lead to pandemics. In the nineteenth century, British physicians documented the spread of cholera pandemics that originated in India. Interestingly, conditions and contaminated water at the Haridwar Kumbh Mela are linked to the spread on at least one occasion.[5] There are other examples tied to more recent pandemics. Some of the first cases of the H1N1 influenza pandemic in 1918 were reported in a camp in the United States where soldiers were watching a football match for Thanksgiving.[6] Almost a century later, H1N1 spread at the Hajj during the 2009 influenza pandemic.[7]

There are also human behaviours that can cause the spread of viruses. Ebola 'spreads through the love' of caregivers who, instead of isolating those who are suffering from the disease, reach out to them. The viral load of Ebola is so high that even dead bodies are infected, prompting the WHO to release a protocol on how to safely conduct dignified burials of those suspected of being infected.[8]

Viruses that cause respiratory infections are not mobile; the people they infect are. On one hand, a virus that spreads well might die out if it originates in a part of the world that's sparsely populated. On the other, a virus that doesn't spread well might continue to cause havoc if it originates in a densely populated city. Viruses need people to behave in certain ways to allow them to spread. We knew this before the COVID-19 pandemic, and it will be true for future pandemics as well.

HIV is thought to have emerged in people from the eating of bush meat in Africa. Rural urbanization led to its spread across Africa. Nipah has emerged from fruit-eating bats in West Bengal and Kerala, India, over the last two decades.

Viruses will continue to cause infectious diseases so long as the catalysts for their emergence exist. Such catalysts include war, deforestation, trade and consumption of wild animals, and agricultural practices that put people near animals. Climate change is expected to accelerate transmissions of insect and waterborne diseases. An intergovernmental report stated the threat aptly: 'The underlying causes of pandemics are the same global environmental changes that drive climate change and biodiversity loss.'[9]

But we are also more likely to identify viruses more than ever. No one had seen a virus or quite knew what one was before the twentieth century. Even during the H1N1 influenza pandemic of 1918–19, there weren't molecular diagnostic tests or ways to check for antibodies. The first immunological tests came in 1929. Just after the Second World War, the ability to grow viruses in tissue cultures became available. Suddenly, we knew what viruses were really like and found them in many places. Being able to grow viruses was key to identifying the H2N2 influenza virus that caused the pandemic of 1957–58. The polymerase chain reaction, which is the key development needed for modern diagnostic testing of viruses, was invented in 1985. Next-generation high-throughput technologies for sequencing genetic material quickly and cheaply became available in this century.

## What must happen for a virus to infect a host?

Humans are exposed to viruses, but very few cause infections to the extent that raise an alarm. Even when infections result, for example, for influenza transmissions from birds to humans, they're usually dead ends. Avian influenza subtypes can often be quite deadly, but fortunately for us, they *usually* don't transmit easily in people. Pandemics are rare events given the number of chance encounters that occur daily between animals and humans.

There are a few conditions that must be met for the transmission of any virus (including SARS-CoV-2) to occur. Let's start with simply getting inside the body before an infection and getting out afterward. The virus has to be able to attach to the body or get inside it. It then not only has to evade the physical barriers of the body, but it also must pass traps like hair and mucus inside the nose (for respiratory viruses) and acid inside the stomach (for viruses of the digestive tract).

Viruses that cause respiratory diseases must find ways to get out of the body. One way they do that is by building up in fluids in the airway of those who are infected and provoking coughing and sneezing. A robust sneeze disperses 10,000 droplets or more, each teeming with viruses. These droplets come in different sizes. The largest ones fall to the ground nearby, infecting only people in proximity. Water continues to evaporate from larger droplets causing some of them to become smaller particles. The smallest particles are a fine plume or aerosol that can remain in the air for quite a bit of time. More droplets are expelled during coughing and sneezing, but they also form in smaller numbers during talking and breathing. Normal talking can release around 3000 particles a minute.[10]

Where do new pandemics come from? Something must happen to disturb a balance. There are changes in a virus that allow it to access humans. And there is a species jump. But there are also environmental conditions for transmission.

There are over 200 viruses that are known to infect humans. SARS-CoV-2 is a new addition to this list, and the number is projected to grow by two to three new viruses per year. Collectively, we need to take measures to track and prevent the spread of emerging viral diseases, which have been increasing due to population, closer proximity to wild animals, agricultural practices, increasing global travel and climate change.

Yet, we should also take a broad view of the virosphere, the entire range of viruses on the planet. An overwhelming majority of these viruses are not detrimental to human health. In fact, some are quite beneficial. Viruses in marine environments are responsible for driving biogeochemical cycles. A large number of viruses infect single-celled organisms like bacteria. A few viruses, known as bacteriophages, are being tested for their ability to kill harmful bacteria in sick people. Other viruses have been genetically engineered to kill cancer cells in tumours.

It is prudent to wonder: if there are so many viruses, why don't more of them infect us as well as SARS-CoV-2 can? The reason we don't have to worry about most viruses is because they are incompatible with our cells. For example, we ingest viruses that infect fruits or leafy vegetables without even realizing it. Because we are so different from the natural plant hosts of these viruses, they can't infect our cells.

The only viruses with any chance of infecting humans are those that spill over from animals. But not all animal viruses can infect us either. It is estimated that there are around 1.6 million different animal viruses in the wild in total. If that's the case, less than 0.1 per cent of animal viruses infect us.[11]

Even if a virus successfully enters a human body, it might not infect people. The virus has to be able to evade the human immune system, which does an incredibly good job of clearing viruses. The virus also must find a matching cell with a special protein called a receptor, which it can unlock.

Once it is inside the cell, it must be able to subvert the biological machinery inside the cell to be able to replicate itself. Most spill-over events are dead ends because viruses can't replicate inside their new hosts. Inside the host, the virus is under severe selection pressure. If and only when a virus can deceive the immune system, and replicate in the host in a manner that it can be shed in large numbers, can it get transmitted to a second human.

Some viruses are readymade in that they only need a few changes to their genomes to be able to recognize specific receptors. These viruses are 'off-the shelf' and ripe for spill-over. Other viruses need to be tailored to fit. These viruses will not be able to infect us immediately but can do so as they evolve over time, while we are in close proximity to their natural animal reservoirs. There may be various rounds of infection and reinfection, while viruses gain the ability to transmit in people better. RNA viruses, in particular, have a tremendous ability to mutate.

But causing a serious public health crisis isn't as simple as crossing over into another species. Scientists visualize the various steps a virus must climb to be able to infect humans in the form of a pyramid.[12] As we go up from the base, there are fewer and fewer viruses. At the base of the pyramid are the substantial number of viruses in the environment that can't cause any disease in humans because they can't infect human cells. At the next level are viruses that can infect humans because they recognize human receptors, but don't spread well. At the third level are viruses that transmit from humans to other humans or from vectors to humans. Typically, these viruses have one or a few cycles of transmission in humans and then outbreaks die out.

Nipah is an example of a disease in this third level. It was first discovered in Malaysia where it was transmitted to people by contaminated pigs. In Bangladesh and India, Nipah is transmitted very differently. Raw date-palm juice is consumed by bats that contaminate it with saliva and urine containing Nipah virus. When consumed, the virus can cause a serious disease that can kill around 70 per cent of the people who are infected. Transmission from one person to another can occur, but these chains are typically short and can be broken through surveillance. A serious outbreak in Kerala, India, in May 2018 was cut short through the valiant efforts of healthcare workers.[13] MERS-CoV is another virus that has a high fatality rate but doesn't spread efficiently among humans.

Finally, at the apex of the pyramid are viruses that transmit well in humans like SARS-CoV-2. These are viruses that threaten lives and become established in populations. HIV, SARS coronavirus and transmissible subtypes of influenza fit in this category. These viruses remain in human populations as long as there are susceptible hosts.

In short, out of a multitude of animal viruses most are incompatible with humans. Only a few develop the ability to replicate inside cells. Fewer still transmit well between people. SARS-CoV-2 is one of the rare few that can infect cells. It also has effective mechanisms for evading the human immune system.

# 6

# Infection

Viruses that infect human cells initiate the process of infection by attaching to specific receptors that they recognize on the surface of some cells. SARS-CoV-2 is much smaller than the human cells that it infects. If an average human cell could be scaled up to the size of a person, one infecting SARS-CoV-2 virus particle would be the size of a small ball. Here's how it infects a much larger cell.

First, it's worth taking a look at the spike. We know what it looks like because its structure has been solved in various configurations that let us see how it appears before attaching itself to the cell and after.[1] And this is important because the spike is essential not only to the appearance of SARS-CoV-2, but also to its ability to infect cells. When we know what it looks like we can also design drugs that stick to it and keep it from working for the virus. We can also design antibodies that bind better.

The virus also contains other proteins: the envelope, the nucleoprotein and the membrane protein. These proteins are not unique to SARS-CoV-2. As I mentioned, coronaviruses also need to make their own RNA 'copier' polymerase and exonuclease 'proof-reader' enzymes to be able to make new RNA genetic material to pack inside viruses.

The spike of the coronavirus is what gives it its sun-like appearance. There are around 100 spikes on the surface of each

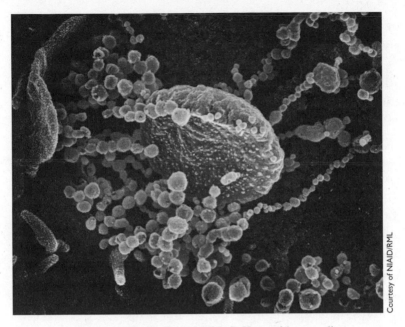

Courtesy of NIAID/RML

Electron micrograph of SARS-CoV-2 and larger cells

virus particle.[2] Each spike is roughly one-tenth of the diameter of a virus particle. And contrary to what's depicted in popular illustrations (including one by the US Centers for Disease Control and Prevention), coronavirus spikes are not ominously red in colour. SARS-CoV-2 does not look like a litchi. In fact, coronaviruses are far too small to have any visible colour at all.

The spike is composed of three identical copies of spike protein attached to one another.[3] Each spike protein is coated with sugar molecules that try to block host antibodies from attaching to it. Remarkably, this virus has picked up ways to fight against host immunity.

Overall, before it has attached to the cell, the spike looks like an extended squash blossom with a long stalk. Quite surprisingly, researchers have discovered that the stalk has hinges that allow it flexibility to scan the surface of cells for the proper cell receptor before it fuses with the cell.[4] This type of flexibility is uncommon in viruses that infect cells in a similar manner to SARS-CoV-2 and is proposed to enhance infectivity.

The tip of the coronavirus spike recognizes and latches on to a kind of protein on the surface of cells called the angiotensin-converting enzyme 2 (ACE2) receptor.[5] A part of the spike called the receptor-binding domain is essential to the process of binding.

The ACE2 receptor is involved in the regulation of blood pressure within the body. Some viruses have figured out a way to use it to enter cells. Not all cells have the ACE2 receptor, but those that do can potentially be infected by SARS-CoV-2 (and by the original SARS coronavirus). ACE2 receptors are found on lung, heart, gut and kidney cells.[6] They're also been found in very large numbers in cells in the nose—an intriguing discovery which explains why the novel coronavirus is able to cause mild symptoms reminiscent of the common cold in some people. The nose is used by the virus as a launch pad to lodge deep down in the lungs where it can cause pneumonia and other complications of COVID-19.

Doctors were curious about the effect of a category of drugs for blood pressure known as ACE inhibitors that work on the target ACE2 receptor and what effect they might have on infection, but right now they believe that these drugs neither improve nor worsen COVID-19.[7]

ACE2 receptors are also found in cells that line the large and small intestines, and as expected symptoms of gastrointestinal tract infections, such as diarrhoea, are also common. RNA from SARS-CoV-2 is found in the faeces of some COVID-19 patients. But overall, actual transmission from the faecal-oral route doesn't seem to be common.[8]

There's a definite progression of SARS-CoV-2 infection that corresponds well with the severity of COVID-19 that is worth discussing. Secretions from the nose accumulate in the oral cavity and head down the upper airway. Infection in the upper airway occurs during the first five days, followed by infection of the lungs.

Cell surfaces inside the nasal cavity contain many ACE2 receptors. Virus particles that are inhaled infect cells there. It is believed that the nose is initially the main site of infection.[9] For some, especially those who are asymptomatic, the extent of infection is limited to the nose.

Presently, we know that COVID-19 is most serious in elderly patients, but the spectrum of symptoms is concerning. Initially, COVID-19 was thought to primarily be a lung disease. Then, we found out that it is also a blood disease. Now, we know it infects many parts of the body.

Why the extent of infection is limited to the nose and mild or no symptoms in some people, and causes serious life-threatening disease in others in the absence of other complicating factors is one of the great questions of disease progression in COVID-19, but it may have something to do with the ability of the body to mount an effective immune response to the virus.

For the cell to become available to the virus, part of the spike protein has to first attach to the receptor. Once the virus has docked to the cell, the viral package which will be used to make new virus particles needs to get inside. To do so, the viral membrane merges with the cell's membrane, giving it access to the interior of the cell. For the two membranes to fuse, the spike protein must be split open by the host's own cutting enzymes (called proteases). This step is crucial for infection to occur.[10]

Once the membrane of the virus and that of the cell have fused, the viral package is now ready to enter the naïve cell and subvert it to make the parts needed to create new virus particles.

How does this occur? As I mentioned, it's quite ingenious because RNA can serve as both the genetic blueprint and also the basis for the creation of viral proteins. The machinery inside the cell that typically makes cellular proteins takes the RNA and makes a large string of amino acids called the polyprotein. Certain proteins known as proteases act as cleavers. When they see a pattern of amino acid building blocks of proteins that they recognize, they make cuts.

The viral polyprotein isn't functional, until it is cut at specific places by a cutting enzyme called the viral main protease. These smaller functional pieces, including the RNA copier enzyme, can now make more copies of the genetic material.

Think of it this way. You have a mechanical loom that can make a designed fabric based on a punch-card program. A large sheet of fabric is made by the loom according to the program. But at the end of it you have cloth that needs to be cut for it to be functionally used from a large piece. This is a very simple analogy, but it indicates why the main protease is so important (in addition to the spike which allows the viral package to get inside the cell and the copier enzyme which allows the virus to make more copies of its genetic material). Without the main protease, the virus can't make functional proteins and it can't spread. As you might imagine, the main protease is also an attractive drug target since stopping it halts infection.[11]

Once all the virus proteins are created inside the host cell, the virus particle is assembled with the newly created RNA genetic material attached to new viral nucleoprotein.

After a new horde of viruses is created, they escape the cell and seek out new cells to infect. During a viral infection, an infected human cell dies because it's depleted slowly of resources by the hijacking virus or because it's killed off by the host immune system. Some viruses cause cells to burst, and others bud out of the surface of cells continuously like small effervescent bubbles.

In contrast the wealth of information on SARS-CoV-2 entry into cells, not much is known about how fully formed virus particles exit cells. Unlike most other enveloped viruses that use the cell's biosynthetic secretory pathway to get out, SARS-CoV-2 and a few other coronaviruses use lysosomes—parts of cells that normally compact trash.[12] In the process, virus particles wreak havoc on lysosomes, preventing them from performing their job of clearing out other invaders and broken cellular parts.

It takes around ten minutes for SARS-CoV-2 proteins and RNA to get inside lung cells. It takes much longer, approximately ten hours, for new virus particles to be made inside the cell. Anywhere from a few hundred to a few thousand virus particles might come out from one infected cell.

Maybe I've watched too many science-fiction films, but I imagine the virus as a tiny round spaceship floating in space in search of a loading dock in a much larger enemy space station, where it can surreptitiously sneak in and cause mayhem. The loading dock has a quite different normal function, but it has been exploited by the virus spaceship. Also, the collision of the virus and the cell is not premeditated, it is random.

But the main thing to remember is that just like the spaceship floating in deep space searching for a place to dock, the virus *needs* a receptor. Infection cannot proceed if the virus can't find a receptor that it recognizes. The virus just bounces around harmlessly and disease does not occur. Cells that have certain kinds of receptors and the right internal milieu for viral replication are ripe for infection.

Specific viruses normally have very *specific* receptors they can recognize. Other coronaviruses recognize other receptors: the MERS coronavirus, for example, manipulates a receptor called the dipeptidyl peptidase 4 to get inside cells in bats, humans, camels, rabbits and horses.

SARS coronavirus also uses the ACE2 receptor as a gateway for infection. What we now know is the fit wasn't as snug for the receptor-binding domains of SARS coronavirus, and so its spike protein didn't latch on to the receptor as tightly. One of the first research articles on to the spike protein of SARS-CoV-2 calculated that it binds the ACE2 receptor at least ten times stronger than the spike protein of SARS coronavirus.[13] How well a virus binds to its cognate cell receptor is thought to correlate with the number and types of cells it can get inside.

After all, it doesn't matter to a virus that we are people. We are an aggregate of cells with receptors it recognizes. A virus is a more likely to jump from one animal species to another that has cells with the same receptor than it is to jump from one cell to another within the same species that has different receptors it doesn't recognize.[14] Receptor specificity is a huge deal for viruses that infect animals and people. A virus is a like a thief going from one house to another with one key, trying to see what it can open with it.

The ACE2 receptor is not just found in people and in bats though. It is found in different animals. Variations between the coronavirus spike protein and the ACE2 receptor in other animals impact how well SARS-CoV-2 infects them. Mutations in the gene encoding the spike protein can enhance infectivity.

*Why is SARS-CoV-2 so good at infecting cells?* The infectiousness and lethality of SARS-CoV-2 virus are what ultimately make unprecedented control measures necessary. One of the first things we learned about SARS-CoV-2, back in March 2020, is that it is much more transmissible than SARS coronavirus.

What makes SARS-CoV-2 so infectious is that it can infect both the upper and lower airways. SARS-CoV-2 infects cells in the nose and throat early in infection. This is responsible for disturbances in smell and taste observed by many who are infected. The virus is most transmissible in this early phase of infection. In those with mild or no symptoms, the infection does not proceed to the lower airway at all.

In those with moderate to severe COVID-19, the virus lodges deep within delicate lungs where it causes pneumonia. From the lungs, the virus attacks the intestines, heart, liver, blood, kidneys and brain. Severe immune responses are seen in many vulnerable people. How does SARS-CoV-2 infect so many different cells in different parts of the body?

One of the most critical early steps in infection is when the receptor-binding domain matches up with the ACE2 receptor.

This lets the virus hook on to the receptor, necessary for subsequent entry. In fact, the pattern of amino acids on the receptor-binding domain of SARS-CoV-2 matches up to the ACE2 receptor much better than for any virus that we've previously seen.

As the receptor-binding domain grabs on to the receptor, another part of the spike protein fuses the membrane that covers the virus with the membrane that is found covering the host cell. For the two membranes to fuse, the spike protein must be cut open. After the membranes fuse, the viral package enters the host cell. SARS-CoV-2 is adept at processing its spike protein for viral entry.

A virus like SARS-CoV-2 uses the host machinery in this process. Before it gets in, it uses host proteases to cut the spike. In contrast with the main proteases that cut the polyprotein which are viral cutting enzymes, viral entry uses *host* proteases.

Coronaviruses that infect humans vary in the number of protease enzymes that they can use to prepare for viral entry. MERS coronavirus has a two-step cutting process that manipulates two proteases. First, an enzyme called furin recognizes a specific part of the spike protein and makes a cut. A second protease, named type 2 transmembrane serine protease (TMPRSS2), makes a second cut. Two out of four human coronaviruses, OC43 and HKU1 (which are responsible for causing colds), also use this two-step process. Furin is abundant in many parts of the body and the ability of SARS-CoV-2 to use it in its infection process may explain why the virus shows up in so many different places.[15]

Quite remarkably, SARS coronavirus isn't known to use furin to infect human cells. Because SARS-CoV-2 is closely related to SARS coronavirus, scientists were puzzled to find that it is able to use furin. SARS-CoV-2 may also be more transmissible because it can utilize furin.

We've seen something similar for other viruses as well. Influenza can have a wide range of symptoms. Most influenza viruses result in mild symptoms, but that's not always the case.

The influenza virus doesn't have a spike protein. What it does have is a protein that acts like a 'key' as well. In influenza this key is hemagglutinin. Occasionally, strains of influenza emerge that utilize furin, and these are responsible for more serious strains of flu.

Some studies have also shown that the spike of SARS-CoV-2 uses a host protein on the surface of human cells called neuropilin-1 to enhance infectivity.[16] Neuropilin-1 is found scattered all over olfactory cells involved in smell, leading researchers to see this protein as a factor in infection.[17]

I'm going to recap the salient details of SARS-CoV-2 infection. Understanding infection is important to understanding the virus. And understanding the virus is crucial to designing drugs and vaccines, and ultimately ending the pandemic. A snug fit by the receptor-binding domain and the commandeering of widespread human cutting enzymes called proteases (including one called furin) to cut the spike protein contribute to making SARS-CoV-2 highly infectious. Taken together, a range of factors explain why the virus shows up in so many different cells and in so many unexpected places inside the body compared to other coronaviruses.

## Receptors and drugs

We can try to keep viruses from getting inside the body by physical distancing and wearing masks. We can inactivate viruses by disinfecting surfaces they infect. But there are also ways to stop viruses once they're inside the body. That's the goal of antiviral drugs. There aren't as many antiviral drugs as there are antibiotics that treat bacterial infections (and that is related to the biology of viruses), but there are some promising leads.

All of the information on how SARS-CoV-2 infects cells I mentioned in the previous section can be used to design drugs and to devise treatment options. Each of the unique proteins of the virus—the spike protein, the copier polymerase enzyme and the cutting proteases—is a target for antiviral drugs. Knowing how a virus works helps us to break it.

There are many ways to design antivirals. We can target parts of the virus or create decoys that prevent it from getting inside cells. We can block the cutting protease enzymes that the virus needs to make functional proteins. We can prevent it from hijacking the machinery of the cell so that more copies are not made. We can tinker with the components that the virus uses so that it makes defective copies that are incapable of exiting cells or of infecting new ones. And finally, we can tweak immune responses so that virus particles are detected, infected cells are destroyed, or viruses can't harm the host.

The concept of preventing the virus from getting inside a cell is simple. If we can stop the 'key' (spike protein) that the virus uses from ever finding the 'lock' (ACE2 receptor) by attaching something else to it (drug or antibody), we can stop the virus from ever infecting the cell. Antibodies that bind to the spike protein form naturally in people who recover from infection and should protect these people from a second infection for some time. These are neutralizing antibodies and they are exactly the kinds of antibodies generated by effective vaccines as well.

Not all antibodies are neutralizing. Not all antibodies target the spike either. In fact, in a study of twenty-two patients suffering from COVID-19 published at the end of July, researchers found that patients who survive have antibodies that strongly target the SARS-CoV-2 spike. On the other hand, antibodies that targeted the nucleocapsid of SARS-CoV-2 are elevated in patients who succumb to COVID-19. This is solid evidence that we want specific antibodies to combat the virus.[18]

Because of the size and instability of proteins such as antibodies, they must be injected: they can't be swallowed in the form of a tablet that enters into the bloodstream. So, there are some limitations to the use of antibodies in a general population or as prophylaxis. But in the absence of an arsenal of antivirals, antibodies may represent the best treatment strategies until effective vaccines are widely distributed globally.

A particular class of antibodies known as monoclonal antibodies has high specificity and shows great promise in treating COVID-19. They are derived from those who were infected with SARS-CoV-2 and have recovered. These antibodies circumvent the challenges of collection and variability of different types of antibodies (some of which might not effectively block infection) of convalescent plasma from patients. They can be used both prophylactically to prevent disease and as a treatment.

When we use monoclonal antibodies as treatment options, instead of waiting for the body to elicit an immune response and build up neutralizing antibodies to infection, we inject them into the body directly. A monoclonal antibody that stops the spike protein presents an effective treatment option for COVID-19. But there may be limitations to availability. It has been suggested that any developed monoclonal antibodies should be first given to those in hotspots of infections such as nursing homes, and to those in essential services who are at highest risk.

A monoclonal antibody developed by Eli Lilly called bamlanivimab was granted emergency authorization by the US Food and Drug Administration in November 2020 for the treatment of mild to moderate COVID-19 in early stages of disease.[19] Another company, Regeneron had developed a combination of two different monoclonal antibodies called REGN-COV2. This combination treatment was given to Donald Trump after he contracted SARS-CoV-2 in October 2020, and received emergency authorization in late November 2020.[20]

These initial monoclonal antibodies are expensive to produce and have to be administered intravenously. All of these antibodies target the receptor-binding domain of the spike of SARS-CoV-2.

Another option is the use of convalescent plasma. In this case, we take the antibodies already formed in someone who has recovered from SARS-CoV-2 infection and give them to someone in an earlier stage of infection.[21] This is not a new strategy, because the use of convalescent therapy to treat infectious diseases has been around for more than a century.[22] A limited study showed that a few patients suffering from severe COVID-19 recovered when they were treated with plasma from recuperating patients.[23] Another well-designed study conducted in hospitals in India found no clinical benefit.[24]

Instead of trying to block the spike from binding to the ACE2 receptor, some researchers have taken a different tact altogether. They are experimenting with creating decoy ACE2 that the virus sticks to instead of actual cellular ACE2 receptors that let it inside cells.[25] A drug company is using this strategy in the hope that flooding the body with soluble ACE2 receptors will fool the virus into attaching to it, instead of to the ones on actual cells. The goal here is to saturate virus particles with something that renders them ineffective in infecting cells.[26] A similar strategy has shown great promise in blocking HIV infection in a laboratory setting.[27]

Yet another approach is to block the cell's own ACE2 receptor so there's less of it for the virus to grab on to. As an analogy, this can be thought of as filling in a keyhole so that the key doesn't work any more. The problem is that the lock (ACE2 receptor in this case) has a biological function within the body. Disrupting the ACE2 could have unintentional side effects.

I mentioned that the virus needs the spike protein to be cut for infection to occur and this is done by host proteases. Removing the cellular proteases that SARS-CoV-2 manipulates to cut its spike protein is another way to design drugs. But here also, we need to be careful. Blocking proteases to prevent viral entry could also have unintentional side effects. Still, TMPRSS2 might be a reasonable drug target compared to furin. Thwarting this protease during SARS-CoV-2 infection may be tolerated by the body.[28]

Recall, that the virus also has a few proteases of its own. Thwarting these proteases poses no such risks since humans don't have them: they're not part of our own cells. Scientists have already figured out the shape of the viral main protease.[29] The next step will be to create drugs that hit this bullseye.

# 7

# Disease

COVID-19 has a wide spectrum of symptoms.[1] Common symptoms of COVID-19 include fever, cough, shortness of breath, fatigue, muscle pain, diarrhoea and loss of smell or taste. Those who have one or more clinical signs of the disease will be tested for the presence of the virus. This is important because the symptoms themselves are non-specific and can be attributed to other ailments such as bacterial pneumonia, influenza and the common cold.

In an early report, the WHO found that 90 per cent of confirmed COVID-19 patients have fever, 70 per cent have dry coughs, 30 per cent have malaise or trouble breathing. Many people who have fever, cough, or shortness of breath may have some other respiratory infection or illness, and not COVID-19. Initially, the probability of having this disease was greatest for those who had travelled to a region where there was an outbreak, or they had been in close contact with someone infected or had travelled: this is no longer the case. Conversely, there are many people who harbour 'silent infections', showing no outward symptoms of disease.

How can we delineate the clinical symptoms of SARS-CoV-2 infection? Those who have silent infections have no detectable clinical signs of respiratory distress. Mild COVID-19

61

is characterized by one (or more symptoms) typically involving fever. Severe cases of COVID-19 have breathing difficulties and other complications, and visible signs on X-rays. They may require oxygen. Critical cases of COVID-19 often require mechanical ventilation since they have acute respiratory distress syndrome.

COVID-19 is a respiratory disease, but complications including blood clots either due to immune responses or viral attack on blood vessels have been observed in some patients. But even after the virus is cleared, usually within weeks of infection, there may be symptoms in people, a phenomenon known as *Long COVID*. In fact, there may be more COVID-19 long-haulers than initially suspected. In a study of patients in Italy, nearly nine out of ten reported lingering symptoms after viral clearance of which fatigue and shortness of breath were most common.[2]

We cannot simply look at the fatality rate to determine the seriousness of disease, because many people will be sick for a long time. Many people who have cleared the virus have decreased lung function and long-term damage to other organs. Loss of taste, smell and neurological effects have also been detected. Inflammation of the central nervous system has been observed. Other reports have indicated that many people have heart abnormalities even after outwardly recovering from COVID-19. There are also reports that survivors of COVID-19 are at an increased risk of deteriorating mental health.[3]

COVID-19 results in abnormalities in many organs in humans compared to other coronaviruses in part due to the ability of SARS-CoV-2 to recognize many different cells that contain the ACE2 receptor.[4] The virus can infect cells directly and can also cause indirect damage from blood clots.[5] SARS-CoV-2 has also been shown to infect the brain and central nervous system.[6]

What is the progression of a typical infection? Virus particles are shed in detectable numbers two to three days before symptoms are observed. Symptoms show up five days after exposure, which is about the time when the viral load is the highest. Approximately 98 per cent of people who develop symptoms do so within twelve days. Infectious virus is thought to be cleared up in about eight days from when symptoms first show up. That's why a fourteen-day observation period is generally adequate to see if someone who has been exposed develops symptoms.

The disease impacts males more than females. Around 60 per cent of patients who are hospitalized are male. The most common underlying conditions for those who are hospitalized are high blood pressure, diabetes, heart disease, lung disease, kidney disease and cancer.

SARS-CoV-2 spreads more easily than SARS coronavirus. In this way, it is easily transmissible like established coronaviruses that cause colds. In some cases, SARS-CoV-2 then lodges itself in the lower respiratory system such as in the delicate air sacs of the lungs. And it is at this second phase that COVID-19 somewhat resembles the original SARS in terms of severity. This is when the virus can attack cells elsewhere that have ACE2 receptors, such as in organs of the digestive system, the heart, blood vessels and the kidneys.

In severe COVID-19, it's not just the virus that is causing serious damage, but also the immune response of the person who is infected.[7] Inflammation, which is usually a sign of normal immune response, goes out of control.

Blood clots have also been observed in patients with severe COVID-19.[8] Blood clots are rare for diseases caused by coronaviruses other than SARS-CoV-2 but have been reported in patients suffering from severe influenza. The precise mechanisms by which SARS-CoV-2 causes blood clots, small vessel disease, COVID-toes and bleeding disorders was not known by the end of 2020, but elevated amounts of a protein factor involved in blood coagulation have been implicated.[9]

Severe COVID-19 progresses to acute respiratory distress syndrome indicated by low oxygen levels and difficulty breathing.[10] Approximately 70 per cent of patients who die from COVID-19 at this stage suffer from respiratory failure. Therefore, monitoring oxygen is important for those with signs of pneumonia. More than half of those who are hospitalized need oxygen.

By infecting a host cell that has an ACE2 receptor, SARS-CoV-2 causes it to sound the alarm to nearby cells. The host cell does this by undergoing a kind of programmed cellular suicide. The signals released are its swansong: they're recognized by nearby cells, which generate signalling molecules called cytokines. Then, these new signals call in the immune force—monocytes, macrophages and T-cells to the site of the infection.

In a healthy immune response in most people, the virus-specific T-cells are attracted to the site of infection where they eliminate the infected cells before the virus spreads. Antibodies block viral infection. All the neutralized viruses and dead cells are recognized by alveolar macrophages, which clear them out. There's minimal and reversible damage to the lungs. Patients with functional immune systems and without obvious risk factors can generate healthy immune responses that quash the virus before COVID-19 progresses to a severe phase.

In a dysfunctional immune response, cells build up in the lungs without being cleared. This causes many cytokines to be produced and they turn on lung infrastructure, thereby causing destruction. These cytokines also circulate to other organs where they can cause multiple organ damage. If there are antibodies that cannot neutralize the virus, they can boost infection instead of warding it off. The sea of cytokines released by the immune system results in something called the 'cytokine storm'.[11] An abnormally low lymphocyte count is a cause for alarm.

COVID-19 severity correlates very well with low lymphocyte count and cytokine storm, which are both consistent signs of an abnormal immune response.[12] Researchers have started to build a core immunological signature of COVID-19.[13] They have found that higher levels of cytokines are helpful as predictors in determining who may need greater surveillance.[14]

## Viruses are quiet visitors

How many people have been attacked by SARS-CoV-2 and have quietly cleared the infection? Antibody tests hint that it is many times more than those who have been sick with COVID-19. But silent infections are not uncommon at all. If critical COVID-19 is the worst outcome, silent infections represent the other end of the infection spectrum.

For many viral infections, there are no apparent damages. Even conditions such as polio are hidden in most people. Polioviruses typically grow in the intestines of those who are infected and are shed in faeces. In about 2 per cent of people, however, the viruses can reach the brain and cause paralysis.

The ubiquity of silent infections surprises people. It shouldn't. In reality, no one is constantly looking for diseases. We are deciding what to eat for dinner, looking at our smartphones, complaining about late buses, scolding children for poor marks, and living our normal lives. We typically worry about a virus only when it makes us sick. In the process of breaking into cells and spreading fast, a virus can trigger the immune system, destroy cells and cause disease. But what happens when an infection doesn't cause disease?

Well, usually nothing: we are often not likely to even know about it. A pandemic is one of the few times when the whole world is prepared to search for infections that don't cause illness in most people, because of how it spreads and the serious illness it can cause in others.

That said, not all viruses cause acute infections like SARS-CoV-2 does. There are viruses which can infect cells and persistently stay inside without killing them; they remain unnoticed by the host, sometimes for years. Persistent viruses can infect or kill immune cells. But often they bear no outward indications. Hepatitis C virus, for example, infects more than 170 million people globally, and causes liver cancer and cirrhosis. Only one out of five of those who are acutely infected clear the infection, while the remaining suffer from chronic infection.

## Testing

In a pandemic we need to know who has been infected with the virus to be able to treat and control spread of the disease. Active SARS-CoV-2 infections are detected through molecular testing of nucleic acid (in this case, viral RNA) and antigen tests.

The most common tests detect the presence of viral RNA. Tests for viruses that cause infections are different from tests for bacteria, because viruses cannot grow on their own. Because SARS-CoV-2 is an RNA virus, a real-time reverse-transcriptase polymerase chain reaction (RT-PCR) is most commonly used, though CRISPR and loop mediated isothermal amplification (LAMP, in short) might result in quicker, though less sensitive tests.

For the molecular diagnostic test, a swab is inserted way up into the nose to collect a sample; however, other samples such as sputum may be used. With the RT-PCR test, if there are SARS-CoV-2 viruses in a sample, genetic material is amplified giving a positive test for the virus. If there are no copies of the virus, or there are so few that it is below the limit of detection, the test comes out negative because there is no sequence to be amplified. A limitation of the test is that it requires a degree of technical expertise to complete.

An issue with RT-PCR testing is that the average physician's office is not set up to use the standard machine at the point-of-care. The instrument required to perform the diagnostic test is also expensive. But reports have shown that samples can be taken at home and can be sent to diagnostic centres. Initially, an RT-PCR test took days to return results. Now, results can be obtained in hours.

Detection of infections early is important to prevent onward spread through isolation, to identify secondary cases through contact tracing and to initiate treatment as necessary. Half of those who were positively identified prior to their death from COVID-19 in two Indian states had been tested less than a week earlier.[15] This diagnosis to time-of-death is shorter than has been observed for many other countries. Testing early is key to saving lives.

A test that a doctor can administer inexpensively which gives results in minutes is a game changer, because the infected person can be isolated and all those who have come in contact can be notified so that they can quarantine. New platforms are letting doctors test quickly at the point-of-care. Some very inexpensive antigen test kits deliver results in minutes instead of in hours.

In fact, there are studies that show that an in-home test that allows many people to test frequently using an antigen-based paper test with a colour change is immensely useful.[16] This test is less sensitive than the RT-PCR-based test, but is cheap. Some experts conclude that the frequency of testing and ability to get quick results is more important in controlling spread than improved test sensitivity.[17]

We watched this play out in 2020. In October and November, Slovakia attempted to test nearly its entire population rapidly using antigen tests.[18] Two-thirds of the population were tested in two days. An additional two million tests were conducted a few days later. The rapid tests unearthed over 57,000 new cases and helped to stymie infections through isolation and contact tracing.[19] Critics pointed to the likelihood of false negatives.

In the United States, the first rapid home-test for SARS-CoV-2 was approved in November. This test can give results at home from a nasal swab in around thirty minutes.[20] At the time of writing, the longer-term implications of quick mass-testing on control are unknown. Nonetheless, the debate over whether to rapidly test more people or accurately test few reminds us of the proverb ascribed to Voltaire that the perfect can be the enemy of the good.

Another diagnostic system with great potential is based on CRISPR, a cutting-edge technology used primarily for genome editing.[21] By September, Indian scientists had developed a CRISPR-based diagnostic system with quick and reliable results.[22] This inexpensive paper-based test received approval for use in November.[23]

How often should someone be tested? Some clinical guidelines for the RT-PCR test call for a patient to be given a clean bill of health after two negative tests forty-eight hours apart. In other cases, a positive result can show up after two consecutive negative tests without any additional exposure. This doesn't mean the person is infectious.[24]

It has been suggested that relying mainly on RT-PCR results to declare someone infection-free would lead to unnecessary use of testing resources and isolation, as there is a shortage of reagents and supplies. In fact, many countries have not been able to test adequately due to rationing of kits. One way to get around this is to pool samples from many people in low-prevalence areas. If the pooled sample comes back negative, no further testing is needed. If it comes back positive, everyone is individually tested.

The RT-PCR test doesn't require the handling of infectious virus, so despite its limitations, it's quite effective. This process is very rapid and highly sensitive, but it's not perfect for everything. The presence of viral RNA doesn't mean there is infectious virus.

The test is sensitive enough that if there is a positive result, we know that the patient is likely infected. A negative test might mean that the virus is no longer present in the patient. It might also mean that there wasn't enough RNA in the sample and it should be tested again. But what about a positive test that lasts for a few weeks? Does it mean that there is infectious virus? For several different RNA viruses, viral RNA persists long after the infectious virus can't be found within the body. It is not unusual for SARS-CoV-2 RNA to be detected even six weeks after the first positive result. This is viral debris.

Here's an analogy. Let's say your spouse calls you from his cell phone while you both are at work. On returning home, you come inside and notice his cell phone, but you don't see him. You could safely presume that your spouse had returned home. But since you don't see him you don't know for sure if he's still around. He may be in the other room. He may also have gone out for a run or a quick trip to the market leaving his phone behind. The phone is a *marker* that your spouse was here, but not adequate evidence that he's here now. Similarly, viral RNA can linger after the infectious virus is no longer present.

RNA is only a part of the virus; it doesn't mean that there's viable virus in the body. That's why the US Centers for Disease Control and Prevention included resolution of symptoms to determine who has recovered. The CDC recommended isolating for ten days from symptom onset or three days after symptoms cleared.[25]

In addition to diagnostic RT-PCR, other tests check for the presence of antibodies to SARS-CoV-2. Antibody tests indicate who has been infected (and may have recovered) in a population. These tests also let us get a clearer picture of how fatal COVID-19 is.

Antibody tests can tell us just how prevalent an infection is, and they can also let us know if someone has antibodies presumably from being infected before. But they didn't have the specificity for personal use in 2020. In a population in which a low percentage of people has recovered and produced antibodies, false positives can throw the numbers off drastically.

Some antibodies may cross-react with SARS coronavirus, but that may not be a big problem in most countries or populations since the virus isn't circulating any more. What we don't know for some of the antibody tests is if antibodies are cross-reacting against other endemic human coronaviruses, which might result in many more positive results. Virtually everyone who had a common cold has been infected with those coronaviruses before, and that might result in undue optimism with respect to SARS-CoV-2 specific antibodies.

# 8

# Treatment

Everyone wants normal life to resume once again. In many ways, the uncertainty around when the pandemic will end has prompted some of my friends to say that they wish that they could be infected with SARS-CoV-2 now, so that they don't have to worry about getting infected later. Uncertainty is extremely difficult to deal with. This same anxiety underpins the desire for an immediate, effective cure for COVID-19. Unfortunately, wishing drugs work doesn't make them work.

Ultimately, randomized placebo-controlled trials will determine which drugs to use. A randomized placebo-controlled trial is a clinical trial in which a set of patients get the actual medicine and another set get a placebo (or water pill). The patients are randomly selected. The doctor is also unaware of the assignment of drug or placebo. These clinical trials are not perfect, but they're a critical step in the evaluation of the safety and efficacy of drugs in evidence-based medicine and for good reason, too.

Let's examine a hypothetical scenario for a moment. Suppose we give a new, experimental drug to 100 patients who have been diagnosed with COVID-19. All of them consent to our experiment and we get necessary approvals for the study from authorities. We check in on the patients as they take the drug every day through its recommended course. At the end of our study, we find that 99 per cent of the patients who take the drug recover. Will we be able to say that we have effectively found a cure for the disease?

Our first inclination may be to look at the 99 per cent recovery rate and conclude that we have indeed successfully found a cure for COVID-19. What we might fail to consider is the natural course of the disease. It is possible and highly likely that 99 of our 100 patients might have recovered on their own with no treatment or simply with standard care *in the absence* of our drug because that number is a reasonable expectation for a rate of recovery in the general population. How will we know the recovery in patients is an effect of the drug? We can't know for sure, and not knowing is problematic.

To dig deeper, let's flip the scenario. Now, instead of giving an experimental drug to 100 patients, if we give them nothing and observe a 99 per cent recovery, will we arrive at the conclusion that a treatment of giving nothing is a cure for COVID-19? Of course not.

Unfortunately, this is what we tend to do in real life every time we get sick. When we take a drug and we get better, we ascribe our getting better to the drug. If we don't get better or we get worse, we ascribe it to the disease.

People don't like to be told that they will get better on their own. We want to take something that will make us better because action is preferable to inaction. We want to be seen as doing *something* even if it doesn't work. But just because someone gets better after taking a drug, it doesn't mean that the drug *caused* it: causal relationship needs to be established.

So, let's now take it a bit further and consider a scenario in which neither doctor nor patient knows if they are receiving an actual drug or a pill made of sugar that looks like a drug. In a very rudimentary sense, we have designed an experiment in which we can compare the effects of the drug against a placebo. If we get similar results for the drug and the placebo, we can no longer attribute successful recovery to the drug.

Trials are necessary, in part, because when we want a drug to work, our intuition clouds rational judgement.

Several symptomatic viral infections resolve on their own without the need for antiviral therapies that treat the disease. Often, we only take palliative remedies that treat the symptoms of the disease, not the underlying cause. When you and I get a cold, we take medicines that help us to manage the symptoms of the cold such as congestion, cough and runny nose, while our immune system fights off the virus itself. But these are palliative, they don't defeat the virus.

It is especially important to distinguish between drugs that fight a disease and those that lessen symptoms or treat other complications. For example, we may take a cough syrup and a drug that reduces inflammation, fever and pain when we get a cold. We would've got better on our own almost certainly even if we had not taken them. Cedric Mims, who wrote one of the most influential medical microbiology textbooks of the last century, put it drolly—a patient suffering from a cold who takes a cough syrup may be cured in two days; otherwise, it may take forty-eight hours.[1]

COVID-19 is *not* the common cold. It is a serious disease. More than 14 per cent of those who get sick may need to be hospitalized; for the elderly it may be even higher. COVID-19 also has a spectrum of symptoms and outcomes. Some people may suffer from long-term effects of the disease that will impact their ability to live meaningful lives.[2] Looking at only fatality doesn't give a full view of the seriousness of the disease. But that is *precisely* why effective drugs can be a game changer during this pandemic. We need a drug to help those who are immunocompromised, elderly, have other underlying diseases, or at high risk for respiratory or organ failure.

Sadly, a poorly designed trial may not tell us anything about the efficacy of a drug at all. We cannot lose sight of the fact that most cases of COVID-19 will resolve on their own, though it may take up to several months to recover. Many children might get infected without even getting sick at all.

If a disease has a 100 per cent fatality rate, in theory, we don't need a controlled trial with a placebo, or no treatment compared to an experimental drug: we can just give the drug to everyone and see how many people get better. For the general population in most settings, the fatality rate of COVID-19 is less than 1 per cent of those who are infected with SARS-CoV-2.

If we give a drug only to a population that is less likely to face its worst outcomes, for example, in the case of COVID-19, to children or young adults, we will overestimate its effectiveness. Finally, we know virtually nothing about how different people may react to drugs. For example, will a new experimental antiviral be as safe and effective in Indian women above the age of sixty-five, as it will be in Caucasian men between the ages of forty and fifty-five? The crucial take-home message is that setting up drug trials is hard, but it is necessary. With a disease in which there is so much variability, we need experts who understand differences in populations and how trials work to design them.

I have heard the argument from well-meaning people that drug trials are fine at other times, but not during a pandemic. I disagree and here's why. Let's say right now you have COVID-19 and are given untested drugs. You get better and think, 'It doesn't matter if the drug helped me recover or I did so on my own. What harm does it do?'

I'll tell you why it matters. When we promote untested treatments, we put vulnerable and exposed populations— healthcare professionals, those who are immunocompromised, elderly, or have underlying conditions—who need a safe and effective drug the most, at risk.

Imagine if the seriously ill had been given a useless pill or told to stand on one leg for an hour each day or clap their hands four times every morning to treat their serious ailment. They might've thought that they'd been given a legitimate treatment, but at best their treatment might've had effects of a placebo.

Worse yet, a broad roll-out of an untested drug (or a vaccine for that matter) to people may not be safe. Instead of helping, a drug may cause unintended, deleterious consequences, going against the dictum of the Hippocratic Oath that doctors take— *primum non nocere*: first do no harm.

## Repurposed drugs

It is well known in the pharmaceutical industry that vaccine and drug discovery take a *really* long time. New drugs typically take a decade from inception to launch, during which time most promising candidates fall by the wayside, often because they don't work as well as hoped, or because they're not safe enough to give to people.

The truth is that every year there are thousands of potential drugs that work in cultured cells that don't make it into humans. You may have seen some of these from time to time in news outlets highlighting the next promising cure for cancer or the next wonder antibiotic. Research in cell lines, in test tubes, and even in small animals very often does not apply to the complex entity that is the human body. How well a drug or vaccine works in a clinical trial is known as its *efficacy*, and that can vary from its effectiveness when it is used in the real world. The path of failed drugs is strewn with concerns on toxicity, delivery to the right cellular target and effectiveness.

Discovery of drugs proceeds like this. Chemical compounds must first show that they work in cells. After a drug or vaccine is found to be promising in cell culture, it is tested in animals, and then in three different trials that test for safety and efficacy before it gets approved for human use. Proper trials must be registered, first to see that they're safe to use and then that they actually work. We can speed up the discovery process, but we can't predict what will happen in clinical trials. None of this is ideal in a pandemic. The virus is already here; new drugs are not. Any drugs discovered through this conventional route will not be immediately useful because they will need to go through months, and likely years of trials.

One way to circumvent that arduous process is to search for drugs that have already been approved for other diseases to see if they work for new ones like COVID-19. The first drugs to treat COVID-19 are drugs that are repurposed from the treatment of other diseases. The advantage of using these drugs is that they have been demonstrated to be safe. The obvious challenge is that they also have to work for COVID-19.

By late 2020, there were thousands of registered clinical trials with drugs repurposed for COVID-19 from other diseases. The problem is, of course, that these drugs were not developed with COVID-19 in mind, and so they may not end up being a 'magic bullet' that will clear the virus, reduce deaths, or shorten stay in a hospital in 90-95 per cent of people who need it most.

Doctors want to help their patients recover and need to make judgements on a case-by-case basis on how to treat a disease for which there is no cure.

Drugs can also get emergency use authorization for compassionate 'off-label' use for diseases other than the ones for which they were originally intended. But ultimately drugs need to go through proper trials in which some patients get the drug and others don't and the effectiveness is compared by looking at both groups. There are cautionary tales we should be aware of where short cuts were taken that eliminated trials altogether.

Ebola is a life-threatening disease that is caused by another RNA virus. During the Ebola outbreak of 2014 in West Africa, in which nearly 30,000 people suffered, chloroquine, hydroxychloroquine and favipiravir were tried out as treatments. None of these was safe or effective. Unfortunately, in a rush to treat a tragic disease with a very high mortality rate, none of these drugs was tested properly in clinical trials.[3]

I mention these drugs for a reason. Six years later, all of these were potential treatment options for COVID-19. Remdesivir was developed for Ebola. We need to  always wait for results from proper trials, and must reserve judgement.

After the first seven months of 2020, there were two repurposed drugs that demonstrated some effectiveness in randomized control trials—remdesivir, an antiviral, and dexamethasone, a steroid drug with anti-inflammatory and immune-system moderating properties.[4] In September 2020, a WHO working group performed a meta-analysis that resulted in expanded guidance to include two additional steroid drugs, hydrocortisone and methylprednisolone.[5] Remdesivir was the first reported antiviral drug for the treatment of COVID-19 as determined by a randomized controlled trial. The drug interferes with viral replication. The US FDA approved remdesivir as a treatment for COVID-19 on 22 October 2020 based on shortened hospital stay among some patients.[6]

However, its effectiveness as a treatment is a subject of debate. In the initial trials, the effect of remdesivir was modest in patients who were seriously ill. There was a reduction in recovery time of about four days in those who got the drug intravenously. Remdesivir didn't improve outcomes in the most serious patients on mechanical ventilation for breathing support, or those receiving oxygen. In fact, results of remdesivir in a very large study showing little to no effect on mortality or hospital course prompted many researchers to question whether remdesivir works at all.[7] Shortly thereafter, the WHO rejected the same drug as a treatment since trials showed it didn't improve survival rates of COVID-19 patients.[8]

Favipiravir is another drug that is thought to be on the same target copier enzyme used by remdesivir, but its effectiveness in randomized clinical trials had not been determined through 2020.[9] In November, WHO recommended against the use of remdesivir based on limited benefit from a large clinical trial.[10] What is becoming clear is that remdesivir, or for that matter any other repurposed antiviral, will likely be ineffective as a late-stage treatment option for COVID-19. Overall, the harsh reality was that in 2020 there were no drugs that worked for all COVID-19 patients in all scenarios.

Antivirals work differently from antibiotics which are used to treat bacterial infections. An antiviral can work on any of the steps of infection but is most effective early in the disease cycle. In contrast, drugs that control abnormal immune responses and inflammation (resulting from viral infection) in certain patients work well later as the disease progresses.

The disease progression of COVID-19 doesn't only involve viral infection and replication which would be treated by an antiviral, but also includes problems with immunity and inflammation in those who develop serious disease. So, a combination therapy with anti-inflammatory drugs in addition to antivirals may, in theory, be effective. Drugs that modulate cytokines such as interleukin-6 are also being tested. In addition, those who have blood clots might be prescribed anticoagulants.

A large clinical trial in the UK found that dexamethasone, an inexpensive steroid, reduced the death rate among those receiving breathing support through mechanical ventilators by one-third.[11] Dexamethasone also reduced the death rate of those on only oxygen by one-fifth. This was the first identified drug to reduce deaths in COVID-19, albeit by modest numbers.

On 2 September 2020, the WHO recommended the use of steroid drugs in patients with severe and critical COVID-19.[12] A meta-analysis of seven trials of three steroid drugs (hydrocortisone and methylprednisolone, in addition to dexamethasone) found significantly reduced risk of dying.[13]

However, use of steroids as anti-inflammatory therapy has a specific usefulness: inhibiting cytokines and carpet-bombing the immune response are not things we want to do when there is a chance of other infections. In addition, the use of steroid drugs has not been recommended for mild infections or early in the infectious cycle.

So far, no positive effect has been found in clinical trials for lopinavir and ritonavir, two HIV/AIDS drugs used in combination.[14] These drugs were thought to block a viral protease enzyme needed for infection. Regardless, the viral main protease remains one of the most attractive targets for drugs.

Chloroquine and hydroxychloroquine (often with azithromycin) are believed to change the pH of membrane-bound vesicles inside cells. The possible antiviral mechanism of azithromycin is unknown. Unfortunately, despite great promise and fanfare, in randomized controlled trials through September 2020 there was no conclusive positive benefit of chloroquine or hydroxychloroquine in COVID-19 treatment or prophylaxis.[15]

A few hospitals in China first reported the use of chloroquine with mixed results. Then, a research letter published in early March (that had been viewed 1.5 million times by mid-June) demonstrated that hydroxychloroquine inhibited SARS-CoV-2 infection in cultured cells.[16] The first clinical results were promising, but were not randomized clinical trials. By mid-March, stocks of hydroxychloroquine, which is also used to reduce inflammation in patients of rheumatoid arthritis and lupus, were depleted in many areas of the world.

The use of chloroquine, hydroxychloroquine, azithromycin and HIV drugs like the lopinavir-ritonavir duo remains controversial. In July, WHO discontinued additional research on lopinavir-ritonavir and hydroxychloroquine after a major trial.[17] Around the same time, the US Food and Drug Administration cautioned against the use of hydroxychloroquine outside of specific settings due to the risk of serious health problems.[18] However, at that time, the Indian Council of Medical Research (ICMR) maintained its recommendation to use hydroxychloroquine as prophylaxis specifically for healthcare and frontline workers based on a case-control study.[19]

Preliminary studies on other drugs such as statins indicate that they may be useful in treating COVID-19.[20] However, randomized control trials are needed. It is unclear if other drugs like ivermectin, which is head-lice treatment with some preliminary results in cell culture, work at all for COVID-19.[21]

Large-scale efforts are under way to identify other drugs that can be repurposed as well. A group of scientists modified cells genetically to see which human proteins coronavirus proteins interact with.[22] They managed to identify hundreds of interactions between virus and human proteins. Blocking these interactions might interfere with the lifecycle of the virus in human cells. They found sixty-six possible target proteins for drugs. Several drugs that have already been approved for other diseases are promising and need to be tested further for COVID-19. One group of drugs might work by blocking new virus proteins from being created in host cells. The second group of drugs hinders the host cell's communication network. None of these drugs has been shown to be effective in treating COVID-19 in people yet. But testing will take less time than for a drug that's made from scratch.

Repurposed drugs will help, but it is important to have a pipeline of new drugs as well. The drugs we have now were created earlier for other diseases. The drugs we will need for 2021 and beyond, including for pandemics of the future, should be designed now. If we create drugs that prevent SARS-CoV-2 from using the ACE2 receptor to get inside cells, block viral proteases, or stop the RNA copier enzyme, these drugs may come in handy for other viruses with similar lifecycles. We need to treat COVID-19, but we also need to build a medicine cabinet for viruses that will emerge in the future because RNA viruses will remain a significant threat to human health.

# 9

# Immunity

When people talk about immunity, they generally refer to the protective ability of the body against infection. But scientists refer to immunity in a broader sense to include all responses of the immune system, not just specific protection. There are two main components of the immune system—innate immunity and adaptive immunity.

*Innate immunity* is a broad and non-specific line of defence that developed in vertebrates much earlier than acquired immunity. It is the first line of defence against invaders such as viruses.

When a virus infects a cell, it triggers the cell and neighbours to sound the alarm through secreted molecules known as cytokines. Sometimes what triggers the system to attack are proteins decorated with sugars on the surface of the virus that mark them as being foreign. Cytokines are molecules used during an immune response to communicate. Interleukin-1, for example, which is formed in cells known as macrophages, raises temperature to cause fever.

Interferons are a kind of cytokine that interfere with the growth of viruses. When some cells are infected, they release these distress signals. These attach to nearby cells and make them resilient against viruses. Cytokines can block viral replication and recruit immune cells to respond to infection. Mutations in human genes and antibodies that block interferons can determine the progression of COVID-19.[1] These antibodies have been found in older males who often suffer from severe COVID-19.[2] The virus can also impede interferons. Viral proteins have been shown to suppress the interferon defence response of the host.

In the immune responses of those who are vulnerable to SARS-CoV-2 infection, and especially in the elderly, doctors often observe an overproduction of cytokines followed by massive inflammation and leakage of cells into the lungs. Airways are often damaged. One of the reasons cytokine storms are common in the elderly is because they have a different immune response from those who are healthy and young. Immune cells spread and start attacking healthy cells and tissues. Blood vessels leak, damaging the lungs. Blood clots can also form. If circulation to organs is cut off, multiple organ failure can result. Up to a third of serious cases of COVID-19 in the US had cytokine storms. Interleukin-6 is one of the cytokines that has been implicated.

Cytokine storms are not a specific feature of COVID-19. They've been observed for other infections, and even some for non-infectious diseases. They can also happen during serious flu. Cytokine storms were responsible for some of the most serious outcomes in patients during the 1918 flu pandemic. In addition, they are not the only aberrant immune responses in severe COVID-19.[3]

Innate immunity is an excellent line of defence, but organisms such as humans have a tailored second line called *adaptive immunity*, which arose in our vertebrate ancestors some 500 million years ago. Without adaptive immunity our lives would be truly short.

A remarkable aspect of adaptive immunity is that exceedingly small regions of variation in an invader are recognized by the immune system. These small structural regions are known as *epitopes*. An antigen will stimulate an immune response by virtue of carrying one or more epitopes. If the epitopes change over time, the antigen might no longer be recognized and won't trigger an immune response. Viruses change epitopes over time by mutation and evade immune responses.

Adaptive immunity is specific and tailored to an invader such as SARS-CoV-2. The immune system also retains a memory of the response for future use against a repeat invader. This kind of immunity is orchestrated by certain lymphocytes which come in two categories: T-cells and B-cells. After an infection, certain virus-specific T-cells attack and kill infected cells. Other T-cells work with B-cells to provide the body with antibodies.

Whenever an antigen enters the body, there are *already* T-cells and B-cells that can recognize it. This is known as the pre-immune repertoire and there are an enormous number of antibodies floating around that have been created for first contact with an invader. They're not present in sufficient amounts to be able to mount an immediate immune response, but the fact that a healthy immune system might contain around $10^{16}$ different antibodies is mind-blowing. That is a ridiculously large number which may be on the order of how many grains of sand there are on the entire planet.

Special cells take apart invaders and present them so they can be recognized by the body. These pieces are antigens, and the cells are antigen-presenting cells. T-cells destroy infected cells and are the conductors of the immune performance. They set up B-cells which can connect to antigens.

B-cells also make antibodies, small Y-shaped proteins that attach to parts of viruses with their prongs. The main kind of antibodies in the blood are IgG. (IgM are another massive kind of antibodies which show up a little bit earlier than IgG, but don't last as long.) Antibodies circulate in blood and other fluids and bind to antigens. By binding to antigens, they block the pathogen's ability to fix to a receptor, and mark them for destruction. Then T-cells attack and kill infected cells.

Strong antibody responses are needed to fight infections and to clear viruses from the body. After infection by a virus, the body produces a lot of antibodies that recognize various parts of the virus. Only some of these antibodies can get in the way of a viral infection by a process known as *neutralization*.

Activated T-cells and B-cells are generally short lived. The exceptions are memory B-cells and T-cells which stick around to remember the intruder. It is worth pointing out that memory B-cells don't make antibodies themselves. When a second infection with the same virus happens, they proliferate and change into plasma cells that do. While the first encounter takes a few weeks to generate sufficient antibodies, the second one usually takes only days. As a result, there are two possibilities: the virus may fail to infect cells in detectable numbers altogether, or it may produce a weaker infection often with milder symptoms that can be cleared more rapidly.

## The duration of immunity

SARS-CoV-2 has infected millions of people, so that even if durable immunity is found to be the norm, there might be an entire range of people who don't have enough antibodies or T-cells.

Does the presence of neutralizing antibodies ensure that there won't be any reinfection with SARS-CoV-2? It is possible that some people may be reinfected.[4] For three of the four coronaviruses that cause common colds reinfections can occur, but it's possible this is because there are mutational variants. What this means is if you get infected with one kind of common cold coronavirus, you might get infected with another strain that has some mutations. We must bear in mind that these viruses have been in humans for a long time; they're established, and so they've had a chance to accumulate many mutations. For SARS and MERS, we never found out if reinfections can occur. The SARS epidemic ended in 2003, and MERS outbreaks are sporadic, so people who have been infected once might not have been challenged or exposed again.

In late August, there was a report of a man in Hong Kong who was the first documented case of reinfection with SARS-CoV-2.[5] The man had a silent infection and showed no signs of COVID-19. Researchers have preliminary indications that reinfection may have been possible because of differences between variants of

SARS-CoV-2. Two hospital workers in India also reported silent reinfections (with no symptoms) three-and-a-half months after their first infection.[6] After a year of the pandemic, out of millions of reported cases, reinfections seemed relatively uncommon.

Usually, antibodies increase two to three weeks after infection. A small study showed that those who suffered from more severe COVID-19 have a greater number of antibodies. And in some people with asymptomatic SARS-CoV-2 infection, the virus clears before antibodies are formed to a level that can be detected. How long do neutralizing antibodies last? For SARS, they were high for a few months and then declined during the following two or three years. Similarly, for MERS, they've been detectable for over two years in recovered patients.

Periodic reports of waning antibodies after SARS-CoV-2 caused widespread fear in the public through 2020. However, a report published in October tracking over 30,000 infections found that most people with mild-to-moderate COVID-19 had robust amounts of neutralizing antibodies for at least five months.[7] Additionally, a large-scale study in Iceland found antiviral antibodies did not decline after months.[8] Another report suggested that antibodies might last for more than a year.[9] This bodes well for post-infection and post-vaccination immunity.

In addition, antibodies aren't the only players in the immune response. Early data indicate those who have recovered from COVID-19 have memory T-cells.[10] T-cells can also have a protective response, which may become important especially if antibody amounts wane.

With a relatively harmless disease like the common cold, young volunteers had been exposed for many years to cold-causing viruses to test for transmission at the Common Cold Unit in Salisbury, UK. Because COVID-19 is potentially a life-threatening disease, there are ethical considerations before we can think of deliberately exposing even young, healthy people (even with their informed consent) to infectious agents like SARS-CoV-2. We can infect cells in a lab with a virus, but really, cells cannot recapitulate all the aspects of a multicellular animal. So, scientists do the next best thing: they infect 'model animals'.

Model animals for SARS-CoV-2 infection include ferrets, transgenic mice modified to contain human ACE2, and non-human primates. Non-human primates are especially useful because they are close relatives to humans in the animal kingdom and have somewhat similar physiology.

Rhesus macaques have emerged as the non-human primates of choice for testing out immune responses and the protective effects of vaccines. Infected rhesus macaques shed virus particles in nose, throat, rectal and lung fluids two weeks after infection.

The first clear indication that getting infected once might confer protective immunity came from these animals. Nine animals deliberately infected with SARS-CoV-2 that cleared the virus subsequently developed immune responses that protected them from reinfection when challenged again with infectious virus.[11] Rhesus macaques are not the perfect proxy for humans, however. SARS-CoV-2 infection is mild in these animals and doesn't span the entire range of seriousness that it does in people.

No experiment has been set up to deliberately infect people who have been infected once, but quite serendipitously, we have some information on the protective effect of neutralizing antibodies from an outbreak on a fishing vessel in May 2020.[12] Three out of 120 crew members (out of a total of 122) had positive antibody readings before the ship departed. None of the crew members had a positive test for the virus. But one or a few of them were presumably early in the infectious cycle (before virus was detected by molecular methods) to cause an outbreak in the eighteen days the ship was at sea. Of the 120 tested crew members, 104 tested positive for SARS-CoV-2, but the three who had antibodies were not among them. Though the numbers are small, scientists think there is a very reasonable possibility that antibodies protected the three uninfected crew members from reinfection.

# 10

# Vaccine

Nearly all experts think even after the current pandemic ends, SARS-CoV-2 will not be eradicated, but will instead remain in human populations. Because it is a new virus that is spreading like wildfire right now, the only hope of ending the pandemic lies in a substantial portion of the global population developing some form of immunity. Such immunity can come from fighting and clearing the virus, but maybe half to two-thirds of the world's population may need to be infected to acquire such *herd immunity*.

Herd immunity in a population solely as a result of SARS-CoV-2 infection would come at a tremendous cost. In 2020, many parts of the world experienced an explosion of SARS-CoV-2 infections. In Manaus, a city in the Brazilian Amazon, the spread of SARS-CoV-2 went out of control. By June, up to 66 per cent of the population of the city is estimated to have been infected; this rose to three-quarters in October.[1] An infection fatality rate of around 0.3 per cent was calculated. This might represent the first natural occurrence of herd immunity in any population. The data underscore the problem with attempting to use natural herd immunity as a strategy for controlling SARS-CoV-2 transmission. The chief concern with allowing the virus to infect everyone who is susceptible is that many millions of people will die in the process of populations obtaining herd immunity.

What we really need to defeat SARS-CoV-2 without the resulting loss of life is a vaccine, or more accurately, many vaccines. Traditional vaccines use parts of disease-causing organisms or weakened, inactivated organisms or their parts to trigger an immune response. They're a way to drill the immune system into recognizing and killing an intruder. Put simply, vaccination is a way to kick-start immunity in the body by mimicking infection without needing to go through disease.

An ideal vaccine provides *sterilizing immunity* in which getting vaccinated prevents infection. That said, a vaccine may not confer sterilizing immunity at all, but offer some protection in which infection would result in a mild disease. People would still get infected and sick, but at much lower rates and likely with fewer serious symptoms. At the end of June 2020, the US Food and Drug Administration provided guidelines for the approval of a COVID-19 vaccine, indicating that a successful vaccine must prevent infection or decrease the seriousness of infection by 50 per cent.[2] Vaccines that received provisional approval by the end of 2020 all exceeded this requirement.

An effective vaccine should do one or more of three things (and an ideal vaccine would show some effectiveness in achieving all three). A vaccine might prevent infections altogether. A more limited vaccine might prevent symptomatic COVID-19. A vaccine might only prevent severe COVID-19. If a vaccine prevents people from getting infected or from infecting others, we can stop spread. If, on the other hand, we can prevent disease and severe outcomes but not infections from occurring, SARS-CoV-2 still spreads (mainly through asymptomatic people), but we save many lives.

Why do we need vaccines in the first place? Well, there are two broad goals of vaccination. On a personal level, we want a vaccine to prevent infection, and if that is not possible, then at least the prevention of disease. On a population level, we want a substantial number of vaccinated people to prevent or slow down onward transmission so that we can reach the herd immunity threshold.

Before specifically discussing vaccines for COVID-19, I want to touch on one other type of vaccines. These vaccines do not specifically target SARS-CoV-2, but instead boost non-specific innate immune responses. Such vaccines include Bacillus Calmette–Guérin (better known as BCG) and oral polio vaccines. There have been studies that have found countries that had universal and partial BCG immunizations had lower infections early in the pandemic, but what this means in terms of guiding vaccination policy is not yet known.[3] Trained immunity from BCG and polio vaccines has been proposed to reduce the prevalence and severity of SARS-CoV-2 infections and is an exciting line of continuing inquiry.[4] But vaccines specific for SARS-CoV-2 will ultimately end the pandemic and are the focus of the rest of this chapter.

When a virus like SARS-CoV-2 gets past the first responders of the innate immune system, it is up to the specialized responses of the adaptive immune system to stop it. COVID-19 vaccines attempt to prevent infections by triggering adaptive immunity. In 2020, scores of vaccines went into trials with the goal of controlling the pandemic: remarkably, a handful had already crossed the finish line by the end of the year.[5]

How do vaccines for SARS-CoV-2 work? If infection with the virus results in robust protective immunity, vaccination should do the same. An essential step therefore is to track natural immune responses to SARS-CoV-2 infection in the body since vaccines will work in a similar manner. An effective vaccine allows the immune system to recognize and neutralize SARS-CoV-2 as it strikes.

A successful vaccine can activate T-cells much like in an infection. Some of these cells activate B-cells that are responsible for antibodies. Other T-cells destroy cells infected with virus in a natural infection. Infection results in the generation of persistent, specialized memory T-cells and B-cells that ward off subsequent infection. A vaccine also similarly elicits *immunological memory*.

When the immunized person is challenged by SARS-CoV-2 in the real world, memory T-cells and neutralizing antibodies step up and stop infection because the response time is fast and effective. If the immune system had a credo it might be the popular saying, 'Fool me once, shame on you; fool me twice, shame on me.'

When a virus attacks the body for the first time, in a healthy immune response, B-cells produce neutralizing antibodies. However, antibodies (which are a type of protein) wane over time. Importantly, and contrary to public perception, antibodies are not the only line of defence in immunological memory. Memory B-cells and T-cells can step up to spur the immune system into action.

A study has shown that SARS-CoV-2 infection results in generation of antibodies in 99 per cent of people.[6] Another study has shown that most mild to moderate infections generate robust neutralizing antibodies and that these antibodies last for at least five months[7]. Recovering patients also generate T-cells.[8] A preliminary study had also predicted that immunity might last a year or longer. All of this is good news: we can infer that effective vaccines are stimulating T-cells and antibodies like in a natural infection.

It is crucial to understand host responses and immunity after infection, because we have not been successful in creating vaccines for all infectious diseases. After thirty-five years of rigorous effort and much promise the world still lacks a much-needed vaccine for HIV/AIDS. This is because HIV-infected people fail to clear the virus as a result of natural infection. A vaccine that mimicked natural host response would be ineffective: it would have to be *better* than the human immune system. Fortunately, SARS-CoV-2 is cleared in most infected people usually within a few weeks of infection as a result of robust immune response.

Reports indicate that COVID-19 vaccines work well in eliciting an immune response similar to that resulting from infection.[9]

## The race for the COVID-19 vaccine

A vaccine for a new disease usually takes more than ten years to be ready to be given to people. In the case of Ebola, which was fast-tracked, it took five years for a candidate vaccine to go into clinical trials. Vaccine development has moved exceptionally quickly since January when the causative agent of COVID-19 was identified. The first vaccines for COVID-19 were created and went through clinical trials in under a year. This was a record and was recognized by *Science* as the '2020 Breakthrough of the Year'.[10]

How was this even possible without cutting corners? Many of the traditional steps of vaccine development were contracted. Initially, many assumptions were made in the development of a SARS-CoV-2 vaccine based on experience with other viruses. Vaccine makers learned from the experience with Ebola. In many ways, the world was fortunate that we were dealing with a coronavirus, because there were vaccine-development plans under way for MERS, another coronavirus. Additionally, many new technologies and platforms were used that increased the speed of vaccine development. This is in contrast with the earliest generation of vaccines for other diseases which used a more passive approach. I'll discuss these technologies later in this chapter.

By the end of 2020, there were multiple vaccines that had gone through the gauntlet of clinical trials and had received provisional approvals for use in many parts of the world.[11] While these vaccines were still in clinical trials, manufacturers had already initiated the process of producing them in the hope that they would work. Two mainstream frontrunner vaccines showed similar efficacy (around 95 per cent) in preventing disease after two doses—a prime and a booster shot.[12] Other vaccines also demonstrated that they worked with slightly lower efficacy.

Fundamentally, COVID-19 vaccines are trying to do the same thing. They hinge on the idea of preventing the spike protein from binding to the ACE2 receptor.[13] This is the key step in infection, and while antibodies can form to other viral proteins, the neutralizing antibodies we want are geared towards this interaction. The virus isn't completely defenceless against antibodies either: it is coated with sugars and tries to keep the crucial part of the spike covered up so that antibodies can't access it.

Traditionally, a vaccine was created from virus that was isolated and weakened or inactivated. The whole virus (or a part of it) was inserted into the body (which made neutralizing antibodies). This is the basis for most vaccines in use.

Within months of the identification of SARS-CoV-2, there were vaccine candidates that used weakened virus, killed (inactivated) virus or pieces of the virus to try to generate an immune response.[14] This is remarkable not only for the speed at which the vaccine candidates were created, but also because they represent so many different strategies.

Without going into the debate of whether viruses are living in the first place, colloquially vaccines with inactivated viruses are 'killed' by chemical treatment or heat. What this means is that after they are injected into the body, they can fire up the immune system but can't replicate inside cells. Whole-inactivated virus vaccines require an additional substance to boost the immune response. This is called an *adjuvant*.

On the other hand, instead of inactivating the virus, a vaccine can also consist of weakened virus to the extent that it causes only a mild infection, while losing all its disease-causing properties. Traditionally, weakened viruses were generated by passing through cell cultures repeatedly.

The safety of inactivated and live virus vaccines is tested extensively since they use actual viruses.[15] Large amounts of virus are required for inactivated viruses. For weakened live viruses, we must make sure that they do not revert to their disease-causing ancestral strains. Again, because a live virus is being injected, extensive testing is necessary to ensure that these are safe for those with compromised immune systems.

An example of an inactivated vaccine is Covaxin which was created in India by the National Institute of Virology of the Indian Council of Medical Research, and Bharat Biotech. Thousands of participants were being enrolled for a Phase III clinical trial in late November 2020.[16]

Other vaccines can be made from protein parts of viruses or virus-like particles, all of which are deficient in some key component present in an infectious virus. Some of these also require adjuvants to fire up the immune system.

A few vaccines consist of virus proteins packed into nanoparticles and injected into the body. These virus proteins are recognized as alien by the immune system which starts to mount an appropriate response. By the end of 2020, Novavax had enrolled patients in Phase III clinical trials for their version of this kind of vaccine.[17]

Another approach relies on creating a 'virus-like-particle' that mimics SARS-CoV-2 but doesn't have any genetic material inside. These are expected to cause the body to mount an immune response, but since they have no genetic material, they aren't infectious.

However, the vaccines approved by the end of 2020 and most of the other candidate vaccines are using platforms that do not require actual virus or parts, but instead use genetic information to get human cells to create the virus parts much like the virus would. These are rapid and safe systems. DNA or RNA is injected into the body where it serves as a blueprint for the cellular machinery to make parts of a virus that are stuck on antigen-presenting cells. The immune system recognizes these cell-created virus parts as being 'alien' and makes antibodies against them. Prior to this pandemic there had been limited experience with working with these systems, although some of these platforms had reasonable success with cancer and other molecular diseases.

Some companies are using the route of a DNA vaccine with genetic material in the shape of a garland. Getting DNA inside cells has been somewhat of a problem. So, a technique called electroporation, which employs electricity to briefly create holes in the membrane of cells, is being used. Once inside the cell, the DNA is transcribed into RNA which is translated into the coronavirus spike protein that can hopefully cause people to generate a strong immune response to it.

But by the end of 2020, the vaccines that had generated the most excitement used RNA. An RNA vaccine skips the first few steps of a DNA vaccine entirely and induces potent immunity.[18] Once inside the cell, it is translated directly into the spike protein which is used by the host cell to build up immune responses. By the end of November, two leading candidate vaccines created by Pfizer and BioNTech and by Moderna that used RNA technology had been shown to be effective after two doses. In December, these candidates were the first two mainstream vaccines approved in the world. The broad use of mRNA vaccines may signal a paradigm shift in how we try to prevent the spread of infectious diseases.

Why are the first approved RNA vaccines only available now? After all, they could've helped us to combat other infectious diseases in the past. Three recent technical advances make these vaccines possible. First, RNA is unstable and difficult to get inside cells. But by encasing it in molecules known as lipid nanoparticles, delivery and stability have been improved. Second, 'foreign' RNA can trigger an immune response (instead of the protein that it helps the body make). But if the RNA is chemically made with synthetic nucleosides, then the immune system doesn't react against it. Third, RNA is 'read' by the host cells to make viral proteins. But before it was modified and stable, it was not read well. The proverbial stars aligned shortly before the COVID-19 pandemic.

RNA vaccines are not without downsides, however. RNA is less stable than many other biological molecules. Enzymes that can degrade RNA are ubiquitous. Even with chemical changes that improve stability, the Pfizer vaccine has to be kept at -70°C. Moderna's vaccine is more stable and can be kept in a regular freezer at -20°C for six months.[19]

The ability to produce and distribute hundreds of millions of doses of RNA vaccines during an *active pandemic* remains challenging. But the good news is that by the end of 2020, clinical trials and preliminary observations following weeks of broader roll-out indicated that both approved RNA vaccines were generally well tolerated. Some adverse effects such as pain at the site of injection, tiredness, headaches or mild fever had been reported, but there were no widespread safety concerns.[20]

The last class of vaccines I want to discuss contain a DNA blueprint inserted into the shell of a harmless virus (usually an adenovirus vector).[21] This is quite ingenious in that it uses a defective virus to deliver a message that will generate antibodies to SARS-CoV-2. These defective viruses generate immune responses but are either too weak to cause disease or are missing the necessary components to replicate altogether. In 2020, AstraZeneca, in conjunction with Oxford University, and Johnson & Johnson were two companies that had enrolled thousands of participants in trials of vaccines that use adenovirus vectors. By late 2020, the AstraZeneca candidate vaccine had shown promising, initial results and was poised for approval for use in 2021.[22]

## How to create a vaccine during a pandemic?

Vaccines that employ many of the newer platforms rely extensively on computer analyses to design sequences to counteract viruses like SARS-CoV-2 using knowledge of coronaviruses and other RNA viruses. They don't require large amounts of virus to be grown, but they do need the sequence of the viral genome. For example, within days of the viral genome of SARS-CoV-2 being available in January, Moderna had a candidate ready to be tested. This would have been impossible even a few years ago.

Vaccine development even during a pandemic follows a standard trajectory. Once a candidate vaccine is developed, it is tested in animals. Researchers find out if the vaccine is toxic. They *challenge* vaccinated animals to see if infection and disease occur. If a vaccine clears this hurdle, it proceeds to human trials. When we first learned about SARS-CoV-2 there were no model animals for COVID-19 and we didn't know if they worked in similar animals. Some vaccines went straight into human trials, while animal models were developed. After these vaccines had demonstrated the ability to either prevent infection or abate symptoms in small trials in animals, they were rushed into advanced stages of clinical trials.

Many vaccine challenge trials started off in rhesus macaques. Inactivated vaccines, RNA vaccines, DNA vaccines and adenovirus vaccines were all administered to these non-human primates (which are very similar to us biologically), after which they were challenged by SARS-CoV-2 through the nose, eyes, orally, or directly into the trachea. After a few days, the animals were tested for viral loads in their respiratory tracts.

What has to happen for vaccines to be ready for human populations? Robust trials have to show a vaccine is safe and efficacious. The first stage of clinical trials in humans, which is known as phase I, tests the safety of the vaccine and whether antibodies (and not necessarily ones that prevent infection) are created. Vaccines are tested for safety and the ability to generate an immune response. Researchers also determine the possible dosage for broader trials in healthy human volunteers. If the vaccine passes this hurdle, it goes into phase II, which checks for immune responses. The dosage and the number of injections that will be administered are also tweaked during this phase. The last major hurdle is phase III. In this phase, the vaccine is given to a large and diverse population. Since vaccines are given to healthy people, phase I and phase II trials may be combined. After clinical trials have demonstrated safety and efficacy, vaccines are approved for emergency use.

Phase I trials are usually conducted in fewer than 100 people, phase II in hundreds of people, and phase III in the tens of thousands. And if designing clinical trials for drugs is tricky, designing trials for vaccines is even more challenging. In human trials, we must ensure that some of the people who are vaccinated have a low background of immune responses prior to immunization. Additionally, we are testing to see that immunological memory remains robust, and infection and serious disease are prevented.

It's important to walk through how vaccines are tested for efficacy in phase III trials. Vaccine trials are different from drug trials. In a drug trial, sick people are given either the drug or a placebo. In a vaccine trial, health volunteers receive doses of either an actual vaccine or a placebo shot. A human challenge trial would involve deliberately exposing these people to the virus to determine outcome, but that's not how the leading vaccine trials have been run. Instead, thousands of people enrolled in trials go about their business as they normally would. Infections that occur later are logged in as 'events'. After a certain number of events occur, the efficacy is determined. We want those who were infected to have received the placebo and not the actual vaccine.

If all the people who are vaccinated live somewhere where the virus is no longer a threat, getting infected is out of the question. The efficacy of the vaccine can't be easily determined. Because of the rapid spread of the virus, this has not been a problem, however. For the frontrunner vaccines, phase III clinical data accrued in only a few months.

Vaccine trials need to enrol participants from various demographics. Clinical trials included people of various races and ages. Yet, through 2020 most vaccine trials had not enrolled children, casting doubt among some experts whether effective and safe SARS-CoV-2 vaccines for children would be available soon.[23] Trials had also not deliberately enrolled pregnant women.

The world will need multiple vaccines. Let's envisage a scenario in which we have a 'menu' of different vaccines created using different platforms but none of these vaccines is perfectly stable or confers robust protection from reinfection. A vaccine that requires two or more shots—a prime and a boost—may confer more robust protection: however, compliance to vaccine schedules is more difficult with multiple-dose vaccines. For field settings, we may prefer vaccines which are stable and do not require freezing at sub-zero temperatures.

The response to a vaccine may also be varied. Think of immune protection from disease not as a black-and-white drawing, but as a more nuanced photo with different shades of grey. A good vaccine should elicit neutralizing antibodies in most people who receive it. The response should be long-lasting. The vaccine may also need to induce not only neutralizing antibodies but also immune cells. If the duration of immunity is short, that might mean that additional doses will be necessary. An ideal vaccine is one that confers sterilizing immunity and prevents infections for a long time with a small dose and with minimal side effects. Such a vaccine should be easy to manufacture, stable and easy to administer to people.

It is invariable that new coronaviruses will jump from other species into humans. We must be better prepared next time. Vaccine programmes for coronaviruses must continue beyond the pandemic.

The holy grail is a super-vaccine that works for many viruses. A really good super-vaccine may be able to cause antibodies to circulate that recognize pieces of the spike protein critical to not only SARS-CoV-2, but also to other coronaviruses. By doing so, it may even offer some protection against related coronaviruses in the wild that haven't yet spread in humans. This isn't a completely fantastic idea. There are broadly neutralizing antibodies that recognize many different viruses. There's been report of an antibody that is able to block both SARS-CoV-2 and SARS coronavirus spike protein, offering some hope for such super-vaccines.

## Vaccine safety

Getting an effective vaccine is important, but a vaccine must also be safe. What everyone agrees is that even in the middle of a pandemic, the adverse effects of a vaccine should not be comparable or worse to the actual disease. So far, with the leading vaccines the news has been good, but vaccines track safety data for years.

Here a few words about safety and efficacy are necessary. There is no such thing as absolute safety because safety is a relative term. Safety takes into account the relative benefits of the vaccine compared to the risks of the disease. Similarly, efficacy is measured in trials, and may vary from actual effectiveness in a larger population. This is because even the best designed trials cannot fully mimic real-world conditions and variability. These points are necessary to indicate that the review of vaccines (and drugs) does not end with provisional approval: as millions of people are vaccinated there will continue to be an ongoing assessment of adverse effects and broad effectiveness.

Vaccines have saved countless lives and are responsible for a higher standard of living. However, among people there may be legitimate concerns with respect to the safety of vaccines. A drug is taken by people who are sick and need it. A vaccine, on the other hand, is given to those who are healthy. Therefore, it is vital to always get it right.

Some researchers believe that ineffective vaccines can generate antibodies that are weak, or worse which can actually help SARS-CoV-2 infect cells, by a process known called antibody-dependent enhancement.[24] Fortunately, through the end of 2020 this kind of detrimental effect had not been shown to occur with any vaccine.[25]

A vaccine given to millions of people must be safe and effective. In 1955, the polio vaccine which contained virus particles that had been inactivated was developed by Jonas Salk. The vaccine took years to develop and was immediately highly sought after. The commercial release of the vaccine was, however, very hasty: the formulation was given to five companies with little oversight. One of these companies, Cutter Laboratories, created and distributed a vaccine that was contaminated with live polio virus which caused 70,000 children to get sick, 164 to be permanently paralysed and ten to die. This is a dark blot on vaccines, but it should also be mentioned that after the tragedy, billions have received polio vaccines and the disease is on the path to eradication.

As noted, vaccines undergo an extensive process by which their safety is examined. Nonetheless, it is almost certain that many people will refuse to get vaccinated. If a large segment of the population doesn't take a vaccine, it is a serious setback to ending the pandemic quickly with less suffering.

## From vaccines to vaccinations

Creating effective and safe vaccines and drugs is only half the battle. There must be equitable access across countries and different socioeconomic groups. There are legitimate concerns that wealthier nations will prioritize their own interests over broader global access. The track record from the last pandemic is not great. In 2009, as the H1N1 influenza pandemic darkened the horizon, wealthy countries purchased supplies for vaccines and low- and middle-income countries were left out.[26] Currently, nine vaccine-producing countries (with only 12 per cent of the world's population) use 62 per cent of the world's influenza vaccines. Inequity in COVID-19 vaccine distribution will be a concern through 2021.

Over the last decade, research and development and manufacturing capabilities have become globally distributed. The best treatments and vaccines against COVID-19 may be developed and manufactured outside traditional centres of pharmaceutical innovation. Cooperation remains a matter of necessity for and within all nations to ensure equitable distribution of therapies.

We should think of vaccines as resources belonging to all of humanity. Companies invest significant resources, both monetary and in terms of intellectual property and expertise, in the creation of vaccines. They need to recoup their expense. But there are broader issues at stake. Should a vaccine maker be allowed to profit from the creation of a vaccine that prevents a life-threatening disease? Who pays for a vaccine created with significant public research funding?

Achieving global, equitable access to COVID-19 vaccines and therapeutics will be difficult. Amid rising populism, governments have resisted multilateral institutions and international agreements. Many countries have responded to this pandemic by turning inward: closing borders, hoarding medical resources and scapegoating foreigners. The first vaccines that have made it through the approval process are a very scarce resource. Demand exceeds supply already. Therefore, the distribution of multiple vaccines ensures that one maker can't monopolize this life-saving resource.

Anticipating inequities in vaccine distribution, in September 2020 the WHO released its vaccine distribution plan.[27] 'The first priority must be to vaccinate some people in all the countries, rather than all the people in some countries,' said WHO Director-General Tedros Adhanom Ghebreyesus, adding, 'Vaccine nationalism will prolong the pandemic, not shorten it.'

Writing in *Nature*, Yot Teerawattananon and Saudamini Vishwanath Dabak spelled out the challenge using visual terms. 'Creating a safe and effective vaccine is akin to striking base camp on Everest—the gruelling climb to procurement and delivery lies ahead.'[28]

The challenge through all of 2021 will be in getting people vaccinated. Vaccines offer no protection unless they are available and people take them. There is a pithy saying that is well-known in infectious diseases research: vaccines don't save lives, *vaccinations* save lives. With all this said, we must applaud the scientists who created live-saving vaccines within a year. There is cause for optimism that effective vaccines will end the pandemic.

# 11

# Parallels

'The past is never dead. It's not even past'

—William Faulkner, in *Requiem for a Nun*

## Influenza pandemics

The woman's expression is grave. She is sick. So is her husband, one of the most influential painters of the early twentieth century. He sketches her. This will be his last sketch. It is dated 28 October 1918. She dies soon after it is completed. He dies three days later at the age of twenty-eight, leaving behind a collection of over 3,000 drawings and over 300 paintings. Edith and Egon Shiele died of influenza during the most severe pandemic in modern history.

When we think of influenza, we tend to think of one disease caused by one virus. There are, in fact, four types of influenza viruses, unimaginatively labelled A, B, C and D. Types A and B are the most serious in humans, and C can cause a mild disease. All known influenza pandemics have been caused by type A, which is further divided into subtypes based on what kind of surface proteins, hemagglutinin (H) and neuraminidase (N) they have. For example, H1N1, is shorthand for influenza type A subtype hemagglutinin 1 neuraminidase 1.

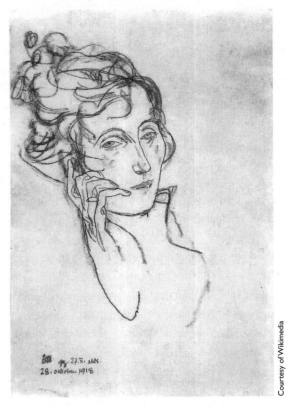

Courtesy of Wikimedia

Sketch of Edith Shiele by Egon Shiele. (28 October 1918)

All the pandemic influenza subtypes have come from different animals.[1] The 1918 pandemic subtype H1N1, also known as the 'Spanish Flu', arose from a bird. The 1957 'Asian Flu' pandemic was caused by a reassortment in a pig, and the 1968 'Hong Kong Flu' also a reassortment in a pig.

A word about the naming of viral diseases. MERS has Middle East in its name. Zika is named for a forest in Uganda. Nipah is named for the village of Sungai Nipah, in Malaysia, where pig farmers got sick. The Ebola virus is named for the Ebola river in the Democratic Republic of the Congo. In the past, viruses and viral diseases were very often named for the places where outbreaks first occurred. However, in 2015, WHO put an end to this practice in specific guidelines to prevent stigmatism of places and regions.

Guidelines put in place in 2015 obviously can't change the association of Spain with the pandemic of 1918. Incidentally, Spain wasn't the first place the virus was spotted. During World War I, military and political leaders of combating Allied and Axis powers did not acknowledge the seriousness of the respiratory disease. The Spanish, who were not involved in the war directly, recognized the contagion after the king got sick and ended up stigmatized with 'Spanish Flu' in the process. The name has stuck ever since.

There is suggestive evidence that the first wave in 1918 originated in the United States. However, it's difficult to ascribe a definite point of origin to the pandemic because it spread simultaneously in three waves through the following year. What is certain is that there were outbreaks in military installations that exacerbated the spread. Much like COVID-19, crowds played a role in the spread. Outbreaks occurred on ships by which troops headed to Europe for World War I.

The 1918 pandemic infected humans and swine almost at the same time because of a new subtype that may not have been seen in humans before.[2] The mortality patterns were quite different from flu pandemics before. Typically, the mortality pattern for influenza is a U-curve, with the very youngest and the most elderly dying. This makes sense because the very young and the old are vulnerable to many infectious diseases due to their inability to often mount strong immune responses. But the 1918 pandemic was drastically different. It had a W-curve mortality, with nearly half of influenza-associated deaths in young adults between the ages of twenty and forty. Why did so many young men and women at the peak of their health die? It has been argued that there is an association with the wartime efforts. But those who stayed at home also perished. Every explanation that I have read for why so many young men and women died is unsatisfying.

The first wave of the pandemic began in March 1918 and spread through the United States, Europe and Asia over the next six months. Illness rates were high, but fatality rates weren't out of the ordinary. The second wave in autumn which spread globally from September to November 1918 was extremely lethal. This was the wave that decimated India. Some countries also suffered from a third wave in early 1919. Three rapid waves within a year were unprecedented at the time.

One of the hallmarks of pandemics of respiratory diseases causing acute infections that make them so difficult to prepare for is that they spread like wildfire. In comparison, the Black Death, which was the scourge of Europe during the Middle Ages, lasted for nearly 300 years.

The singular feature of the 1918 pandemic that keeps it in public memory over a century later is just how deadly it was; there was no virology at the time to accurately pinpoint those who were infected, so case counts are based on symptoms of infection. But conservative estimates are that around 40 million died. An estimate at the other end of the range is that as many as 100 million people might've perished from influenza and associated complications. India bore a heavy burden with a whopping 14 million or more dead.

Why did relatively more Indians die compared to people in other countries? There are no good answers, only intuitive theories.[3] At the time, India was a conglomeration of many densely populated rural areas under colonial rule. Approximately 75 per cent of people lived under the British Crown and 25 per cent in princely states. The country suffered periodically from outbreaks of cholera, typhoid, plague, smallpox, TB and other infectious diseases. Malnutrition was high. Famines occurred occasionally.

H1N1 arrived in India in Mumbai, likely through transport routes. Then it fanned out by train to the rest of the country.

When the virus hit, no one could grasp the scale of the crisis. Britain was preoccupied with war. Mahatma Gandhi was one of those who fell sick. A fuller study of the economic, healthcare and political factors that made India one of the worst affected nations is lacking, but necessary.

But the virus was not only deadly, it was also transmissible. Influenza, both of the seasonal variety and the pandemic one, spreads very quickly. Most patients with symptoms recover after a fever of three to five days. Sometimes complications can arise leading to worse outcomes.

Why was the virus so deadly? It wasn't simply due to destruction of lungs. The complete genome of the strain has been sequenced. Some of the genes have been genetically engineered into other influenza strains to study effects, and these strains have been used to infect animals to see what happens. It is possible that the 1918 strain flu contained an enzyme that disturbed the functioning of immune system cytokines, namely, interferons. As we've observed for COVID-19, for the 1918 H1N1 influenza pandemic, there was a hyperactive immune response and inflammation. Yet, there is still much to learn about the lethality of the H1N1 strain and what made it so dangerous in people.

During that pandemic, many patients were also infected by bacteria at the same time and suffered from mixed pneumonia. Because there were no antibiotics, other bacteria infected young healthy people. There were insufficient beds to treat patients, mechanical respirators and supplemental oxygen were not available, and the world was at war. In addition, leaders played down the threat of the virus. It was a complete failure on all fronts.

To this day, the 1918 pandemic represents the worst observed modern pandemic. Even with modern antiviral and antibacterial drugs, vaccines and prevention, the return of a pandemic virus with the disease-causing ability of the H1N1 influenza virus of 1918 would kill millions of people worldwide. But it is not the worst that is *possible*. The estimated case-fatality rate of H1N1 during that pandemic is 2.5 per cent which is twenty-five times higher than that of the seasonal flu, but still low compared to some other diseases. For example, a pandemic virus with the deadliness of H5N1 would cause proportionately more deaths.

The second pandemic of the twentieth century began in 1957 with the appearance of an H2N2 subtype in East Asia. As we've seen for most pandemics, the precise location where influenza originates is often unknown because of the speed with which pandemic viruses spread. Unlike in 1918, there were virological tools: the virus could be isolated and grown on cells in the lab. There was a diagnostic test for the subtype.

The mortality of H2N2 influenza in 1957 plotted as a typical U-curve seen with seasonal influenza, with the very young and the old most likely to die. The virus attacked those in school and at work more than those who stayed at home; but killed more elderly. The virus spread in the southern hemisphere first and then in the northern hemisphere. The overall impact was only one-tenth of that observed in 1918-19.

Italy was hit hard, reminiscent of the COVID-19 pandemic in that country in February 2020. The actor Ingrid Bergman was ill in her apartment in Rome. An American passenger ship arrived in San Francisco from Japan with nearly everyone on-board sick or recovering.

It is estimated that over 1 million people died in the H2N2 pandemic of 1957. But the fact that a vaccine was created quickly saved many lives. The pandemic ended after several waves in which people became immune over three years.

The third and last influenza pandemic of the twentieth century occurred in 1968 with the emergence of an H3N2 virus, also referred to as Hong Kong influenza. This was a 'hybrid' pandemic strain because only one of the surface glycoproteins, the hemagglutinin H3, was unique for the population. The neuraminidase N2 had been present in the pandemic subtype of 1957. This hemagglutinin was not completely unknown in humans, since it is thought to have been part of the signature of the influenza virus that caused an earlier pandemic. The H3N2 influenza virus was detected in September 1968, but deaths only started to peak in December. This virus stuck around for a while, returning in 1970 and 1972 but wasn't as deadly as the viruses of 1918 or 1957. It's estimated that the virus was probably about half as deadly as the pandemic influenza virus of 1957. It's also true that improved medical care, antibiotics for secondary bacterial infections and more advanced care limited deaths.

Flash forward to 2009. The H1N1 pandemic of 2009 is one that I distinctly remember because I lived through it and wrote about it.[4] Flu-like respiratory illness had first been reported in a town in Veracruz, Mexico, in mid-February. A five-year-old boy, Edgar Hernandez, is believed to be the first known case.[5] He survived and is commemorated by a statue in his hometown in Mexico. Because it was a similar strain to the 1918 virus and because initially it was thought to be very deadly, measures were taken globally to prevent spread.

Young people had little immunity, but those over sixty had antibodies possibly from an earlier virus attack. Approximately 80 per cent of deaths occurred in people younger than sixty-five. Seasonal flu vaccines offered only marginal protection. A vaccine was available, but only after the first wave was gone.

Though the 2009 flu pandemic primarily affected children and young and middle-aged adults, the impact of the virus on the global population during the first year was less severe than that of previous pandemics. It is possible that less than 600,000 people worldwide died in the first year that the virus circulated. Overall, the pandemic subtype might have been less deadly than the seasonal influenza virus in circulation at the time. On 10 August 2010, the WHO declared an end to the global 2009 H1N1 influenza pandemic. However, 2009 H1N1 didn't vanish: it's one of the seasonal flu viruses that causes sickness and death in people across the world.

Why didn't the 2009 H1N1 influenza subtype create a greater splash? The 2009 H1N1 influenza strain was highly transmissible, but not very deadly. Many nations felt that the pandemic was grossly overestimated initially in terms of severity.[6] Changes were made to pandemic preparedness processes considering the 2009 experience.

Our experience with previous influenza pandemics should've prepared us for the next pandemic. Only, it wasn't an influenza strain at all this time.

## Where do pandemic subtypes of influenza come from?

Influenza viruses are like coronaviruses in that both are enveloped RNA viruses.

Like coronaviruses, influenza viruses also encode for an RNA-dependent RNA polymerase copier enzyme, but influenza viruses lack specific proofreading activity. So, influenza viruses make a lot more mistakes than coronaviruses. Over the length of its genome, SARS-CoV-2 accumulates an average of about one to two mutations per month which is about one-fourth to one-half the rate of mutation for influenza.

RNA viruses can swap entire tracts of their genetic material to create a new 'fusion' virus by a process called recombination. Recombination occurs when two different viruses infect the same cell at once. The progeny inherits genetic pieces from each of the 'parent' viruses, and it's the closest to sexual reproduction in viruses.

Like coronaviruses, influenza virus is also an RNA virus that can undergo recombination, and it's thought that this process results in strains with pandemic potential. However, unlike coronaviruses which have one long, intact RNA strand as genetic material, influenza has genetic material in eight pieces. What this means is that sometimes when two different influenza viruses infect the same cell, their offspring can pick up different pieces.

Influenza viruses mainly infect the upper respiratory tract. They cause respiratory infections leading to influenza disease, or what is known as the flu. We all know the symptoms of mild flu— fever, cough and muscle pain. The disease is typically self-limiting and lasts about a week. Most people develop a robust immune response to seasonal flu strains and antibodies to specific types of hemagglutinin and neuraminidase. But even the seasonal influenza can be a serious disease in the young and the elderly. The young don't yet have antibodies from earlier infections with similar strains, and the elderly don't have robust immune responses any more.

When people refer to the flu what they're referring to is the relatively mild seasonal (or annual flu) that comes up every year, and not the pandemic influenza that shows up every few decades. Seasonal flu is a part of life.

Every year or so there's influenza with seasonal variation, starting around October or November and then ending around March in the northern hemisphere. Every year, there is immunity built up in a population, but the flu picks up mutations that cause something called *antigenic drift*. Think of it as being a slight drift that causes a blur in the memory of the immune system, resulting in infections leading to a mild form of disease. These arise from an accumulation of single *point mutations* or a few of them at a relatively reasonable frequency. That's one reason we need to make flu vaccines every year.

But, in addition to antigenic drift, we also must talk about how new subtypes of influenza arise through major change, known as *antigenic shift*. Influenza viruses exist in a wide variety of species and they have different antigenic properties. There are eighteen different hemagglutinin types. These variations are present in influenza viruses that infect mammals and bird species. And every so often, new influenza viruses emerge with hemagglutinins for which humans have no immunity. If these subtypes can spread well in humans, we have the recipe for a disastrous pandemic.

Antigenic shift results in a virus that the immune system perceives as new. This typically occurs every few decades.

So how do pandemic subtypes of influenza typically originate? Pigs are what virologists call 'mixing vessels'. Pigs can get infected with porcine influenza of course, but they can also get infected with avian influenza from birds such as ducks and chickens, and human influenza from people. Avian subtypes of influenza are very deadly in people, but so far, they've not been known to replicate well in people, so human-to-human chains of transmission are typically short.

Pigs swap pieces of different influenza viruses back and forth. When two different viruses infect the same cell, the genetic material mixes and a completely new virus emerges. This might be happening very frequently, but only those that confer some selective advantage in terms of greater transmission or other traits get selected. The influenza virus that originates in a pig is now ready to infect people readily.

Agriculture in a mixed setting with a lot of pigs, ducks and chickens as well as humans in proximity tends to exacerbate the situation.[7] Subunits from birds get mixed in pigs and transferred on from the pig reservoir. And suddenly, we have an entirely new configuration of an antigen on the viral surface. The existence of influenza viruses in poultry (mainly ducks), the closeness of people to animals and butchering of different animals in live markets all contribute to East Asia being a hotspot for pandemic influenza subtypes, though at least one pandemic strain, H1N1 2009, emerged out of Mexico.

What is extraordinary is that there are parallels in the origin of pandemic strains of influenza in pigs to what we think may have occurred for SARS coronavirus and possibly SARS-CoV-2. Like influenza viruses, coronaviruses are also capable of picking up pieces of genetic material from one another.

# 12

# Prevention

## People are virus factories

What does a factory do? It spews out smoke and a lot of toxic compounds, some of which we can't see. It helps to visualize people as factories that are emitting viruses. If they are infectious, but don't feel sick, they may be shedding viruses while breathing and talking without knowing it themselves.

In order to get infected, a certain minimum number of virus particles must get inside your body. We will get to what that number might be for SARS-CoV-2 infections later, but suffice it to say that this process can happen at once or over an extended interaction. If you visualize someone as being infected and shedding virus particles at a constant rate by breathing or talking loudly, the closer you are to them, the more you are likely inhale virus particles. If both of you are wearing masks, the number of virus particles that either of you is exposed to is reduced. If your interaction time is short, exposure time is likewise reduced.

When infected people cough and sneeze, they release many virus particles through droplets, but there is a basal level of virus particles that are exhaled when an infected person is breathing. Speaking increases this rate by about ten times. Singing is, of course, a more forced expulsion of air and causes an even greater amount of virus particles to be released.

In July 2020, at the behest of over 200 experts, the WHO agreed to review their guidance on how SARS-CoV-2 spreads to include transmission via small aerosols. Prior to that they had confirmed spread through *respiratory droplets*, which are small particles in the range of 5000 to 20,000 nanometres. A nanometre is one millionth of a millimetre.

Aerosols are smaller than droplets and under 5000 nanometres. Droplets undergo gravitational settling: they fall to the ground and contaminate surfaces they fall on. Aerosols, which are smaller, linger and are affected by air currents. When droplets are expelled, they start to evaporate. Some of them invariably become small enough to be carried by air currents as aerosols.

A paper in *Science* compared aerosols to cigarette smoke.[1] If you can smell the smoke from someone smoking at a certain distance, you can get a sense of how far aerosols can travel. But the further away you are from an infected person, the fewer virus particles you stand a chance of breathing in. In the outdoors, the plume is diluted.

Human coronaviruses and influenza viruses had all been found in both droplets and aerosols before this pandemic. Aerosol formation of virus-laden faeces of a person who was infected in an apartment complex caused the most serious outbreak of SARS in Hong Kong in 2003 in which over 300 people were infected. SARS coronavirus particles had also been shown to be emitted while speaking. One minute of loud talking generated around 1000 virus-laden aerosol particles. That transmission by aerosols was likely, where secondary cases were not sitting in proximity to an infected individual, was evident from one case of transmission on an airplane during the H1N1 influenza pandemic of 2009. Normal talking by someone infected by SARS-CoV-2 can generate around 3000 aerosol particles. In the early stages of infection each aerosol particle has been estimated to contain 250 virus particles.[2] Multiplying these two numbers gives us 750,000 virus particles each minute.

During this pandemic, it became clear that people who were infected but not sick were spreading the disease silently. A significant proportion of spread of SARS-CoV-2 is by asymptomatic carriers who can spread virus-laden particles as aerosols from anywhere between three to twelve days. Someone who has a silent infection is not sneezing or coughing large droplets, so it became natural to suspect that they are spreading the virus by means such as by speaking, breathing, or singing. Air samples collected from Wuhan and from isolation rooms in hospitals in the United States had the tell-tale signs of SARS-CoV-2. Given the rapid spread of SARS-CoV-2 on the *Diamond Princess* cruise ship, it was possible to surmise that airborne transmission was occurring. Since then the signatures of the virus have been detected in ducts of indoor air-conditioning systems and other places in buildings where droplets which fall due to gravity should not be found.

The smoking gun that established airborne spread was a report of a choir practice in Washington on 10 March 2020.[3] After a two-and-a-half-hour choir practice, a symptomatic patient infected as many as fifty-two people of which two died. It's almost certain that singing contributed to the expulsion of aerosols. This situation is not unique to the spread of SARS-CoV-2. Singing in groups with people who suffer from respiratory tuberculosis has also been known to spread TB germs.

Sick people are less likely to talk or sing a lot, but those who harbour germs but don't know it because they're not sick can spread infections to many. Researchers have looked at droplet formation from different consonants for other respiratory diseases: more are formed when words with 'f', 'p', 's', and 't' are spoken. However, the relevance to SARS-CoV-2 spread is unknown.

Faecal-oral transmission of coronaviruses is common among bats that harbour coronaviruses but doesn't seem to be a major means of spread of SARS-CoV-2 among humans. There have been reports that flushing toilets with the lids open releases an aerosol, and it is conceivable that forced flow of water may also do the same with a squat latrine.[4] SARS-CoV-2 RNA has been detected in faecal matter of patients with COVID-19 and in sewage and wastewater, but actual infections from faecal matter had not been persuasively documented among the millions of reported cases in 2020.[5]

## How effective are individual measures in stopping transmission?

During a pandemic some of the most practical concerns are day-to-day. How can I protect myself and my loved ones? How can I accurately assess my own risk and that of family members?

Biological characteristics of SARS-CoV-2 come into play in determining risk. There are also aspects of surroundings, such as environmental factors. What is less well known is what predisposes one person to infection and serious COVID-19 more than another person of the same age and health status. As we learn more about innate factors that partially determine susceptibility and disease progression in different people, we will be able to answer this question better.

SARS-CoV-2 is a new virus, but it didn't come from outside the solar system. It has novel features, but in many aspects, it is representative of other viruses causing acute respiratory infectious diseases that have been studied for over a century. SARS-CoV-2 manifests in many additional ways because of its ability to infect many different cells, but there are other coronaviruses that routinely infect people. There are also other viruses such as influenza that have an outer layer of lipid.

Like many other people, I've come across an endless stream of questionable prevention techniques and cures. They are typically easy to dispel. When someone offers an untested drug as a cure, it is prudent to ask *how* it is expected to treat COVID-19 or lessen its symptoms. While the details of mode of action of a cure might not be known initially, there must be a plausible explanation. Miraculous claims should be treated with scepticism. Disinfectants should never be ingested. Drinking a lot of alcohol or water will not inactivate a virus lodged in a person's respiratory tract. Eating meat will not transfer a virus that is spread now from one human to another; conversely, vegetarians are not less likely to get infected. There's no way to shine ultraviolent light on infected cells to kill the virus. Common sense is the best preventative measure.

## How can I reduce the risk of infection?

When we ask, 'does a measure work in stopping infection?' we expect the answer to be in the form of a 'yes' or 'no'. But often the answer is not that simple. We must consider each measure, how it prevents spread, and the difficulty in implementing it. Then we must consider layering as many as we can together. In really wintry weather we wear layers of clothing because each provides a certain level of warmth that cumulatively causes us to feel comfortable. Remove the jacket or the sweater, and we are exposed a little bit more.

Multiple measures tend to work best in reducing risk. A research article found that increasing the physical distance from close contact to over 1 metre between people reduced the chance of infection or transmission from 12.8 per cent to 2.6 per cent.[6] The use of facemasks reduced it from 17.4 per cent to 3.1 per cent. And wearing eye protection reduced it from 16.0 per cent to 5.5 per cent. While the chance of infection might change in different situations, this study indicates that these measures are effective in significantly reducing personal risk

Personal measures that should be used at all times include staying at home when ill, covering mouth when coughing, hand-washing and physical distancing. Others may be situation specific, such as the use of masks outside of the house and working from home if the option exists and there is a cluster of infections in the vicinity.

Someone who is young and does not have a known high-risk condition is at a lower risk for an adverse outcome compared to someone who is older and has known complicating conditions such as heart disease. Similarly, someone who is working in a building where other people have been infected has a greater occupational risk than someone who is working from home. Individual circumstances determine the stringency of the measures someone might take.[7] But unless you live in a bunker with your own supply of food, there is practically no way to reduce your risk of getting infected to zero. This is a fact. However, the relative chance that you will get infected if you take specific measures can go down appreciably.

Shortly after I joined graduate school in a microbiology department in 2001, I started working in a lab. Before I could handle radioactive materials and hazardous chemicals required in standard molecular biology techniques, I had to undergo training on how to handle them safely. I learned the important 'As Low As Reasonably Achievable' principle (better known by the acronym, ALARA).[8] Before every experiment, I set up safe zones, wore lab coats and gloves, and used shields and facemasks. I exposed myself to the minimum amount of radiation *reasonably* possible by minimizing the amount and time I handled radioisotopes.

Now, going to a grocery store is very different from working with phosphorus-32 in a lab, but during a pandemic, the ALARA principle applies to our activities. We want to reduce potential exposure to the virus by restricting movements outside the home, having a plan for such sojourns and spending no more time than necessary. We mustn't lose sight of being reasonable, and there's no universal definition of reasonable because it depends as much on a person's risk tolerance as it does on empirical risk.

It is important to remember that just because someone can theoretically get infected in a certain way doesn't mean that it will happen. Let me explain. Right now, I may be typing away blissfully near a whirring fan. Can the fan fall on my head? If I'm sitting beneath it, sure. Will it fall on my head? That depends on a lot of factors, but based on what I know right now, it is not a reasonable risk. The risk may change in the future, but the chance is low and acceptable to me.

Some people who take precautions will get infected and others who take none won't. It should be obvious to us that our goal is not to remove all risk. That is impossible for most of us who must interact with other humans and human-touched objects from time to time. The purpose is to reduce risk to reasonable levels.

Typically, low-risk activities include opening packages (including ones that contain books like this one), getting carryout food from restaurants, grocery shopping and going for a walk or a run. Having dinner at someone else's house, going to the beach, sending children to school, or working in an office for a week carries a moderate amount of risk. The risk for someone who is working a shift inside a store is greater than the casual shopper, even if the overall risk for both is low. Watching a film in a theatre, going to a sporting event in a stadium, participating in a religious event with hundreds of others or attending a wedding carries greater risk.

Getting direct evidence of transmission is extremely hard. For a relatively mild disease like the common cold, volunteers were exposed over years at the Common Cold Unit. This probably won't happen for COVID-19 because it is a more serious disease. We have experiments on transmission in animals. Most infections occur from people to other people in indoor settings. There are other ways of getting infected such as from surfaces, but they carry a very low risk.[9]

## Social distancing

What exactly is social distancing? WHO called it staying at an arm's length from another person who might be infected to prevent spread of a respiratory infectious disease, or in numerical terms, 1 metre apart (the official advisory). Some countries, including India, China, Denmark and France, adopted WHO guidelines. The CDC recommended avoiding crowds and 'maintaining distance (approximately six feet or two metres) from others when possible'. The UK went with two metres. Australia, Germany, Italy and Spain recommended 1.5 metres. Why was there so much confusion and disparity between countries on this important concept?

The truth is none of these advisories was based on any research on SARS-CoV-2 and how it spreads. These advisories dated back decades, and did not consider the possibility of spread of aerosols, a likely manner of transmission in certain situations such as crowded bars with a lot of loud talking. As a rule of thumb, at least two metres (further apart is better) may be advisable indoors where there is a greater chance of aerosols forming. Aerosols, formed from breathing, talking and singing contain fewer virus particles than droplets, but travel farther and linger longer. Outdoors, when there are no crowds, aerosols are diluted faster. But even a forcefully expelled sneeze or cough is unlikely to stay within a one-metre zone. It should be noted that aerosols will dilute the further out we are from their source.

A model utilizing mobile-phone data of nearly 100 million people in major US cities to track movements suggest that super-spreader events in crowded venues like restaurants, cafes, gyms and hotels might be responsible for most SARS-CoV-2 infections.[10] Limiting occupancy in indoor settings (and spending less time in crowded areas) can reduce infections.

## Masks for all

How can we personally limit the spread of SARS-CoV-2? Research has shown that the spread of SARS-CoV-2 from one person to another via respiratory droplets and aerosols is many times more prevalent than spread from surfaces and objects contaminated with the virus.

It makes sense therefore to filter virus particles so they can't leave or get inside the body. The use of facemasks and other face coverings has been estimated to have reduced infections in Wuhan, China, parts of Italy and New York City through mid-2020. Facemasks are cheap, effective when used properly and can be layered as a measure with handwashing, social distancing and eye protection to reduce risk of infection.

It is intuitive to assume a facemask protects the wearer. A mask is probably more effective in preventing infections by stopping droplets and aerosols in the outward direction, provided it does not have a valve that opens. Facemasks can stop virus-laden particles released by breathing and talking from getting out. Given the significant transmission by those who are infected but don't know it, protection in both directions is a necessary safeguard.

The commercial N95 respirator is the best in terms of filtration among those that are routinely used by the public, but surgical masks and cloth masks are also effective to a certain extent. There is evidence that a well-constructed cloth facemask can reduce both droplet and aerosol transmission for SARS-CoV-2 just as it does for other respiratory infectious diseases.

Cloth facemasks with larger pores and lower thread counts act primarily as physical barrier. But physical barriers can be augmented. N95 respirators and cloth facemasks with multiple layers of different cloth are more effective in providing electrostatic barriers that can block smaller particles.

Facemasks alone are not capable of completely removing the threat of spread, but they might reduce it, especially by asymptomatic and pre-symptomatic people in situations where social distancing is not possible such as indoors, especially in shopping centres, clinics, busy footpaths, public transportation, schools and offices that have poor circulation. The key is that they must be used with the assumption that everyone is infected.

The goal of wearing facemasks is not to stop all transmission but to stop it as much as possible. In parts of Asia, facemasks are available year-round in pharmacies and are worn for protection and out of politeness. This may become a global trend even after the pandemic ends.

Some countries solved the problem of equitable distribution of surgical facemasks with great ingenuity. In South Korea, for example, people were able to buy a limited number of masks from pharmacies based on specific days of the week. Control of the process ensured there was never a prolonged shortage. Taiwan had a similar process for distribution. This prevented hoarding and kept prices down.

In many countries, there was unnecessary delay in the implementation of masking also because of the propensity of humans to think in terms of binaries of whether masks work or don't, and the resulting opaque communications from public health officials. It is true that facemasks vary in their type and ability to filter out virus-laden droplets and aerosols. Effectiveness also depends on the length of use, and proper fitting and removal. But masks are also minimally disruptive, and they need not impede breathing during normal activities in healthy people to be effective.

Even when the impact is modest, the possible benefit outweighs the potential harm. A single layer of a T-shirt, scarf, sweatshirt, or towel is efficient in blocking anywhere from 10 per cent to 40 per cent of saline aerosols mimicking viral aerosols. Adding layers adds to efficiency. A tea-towel fabric with two layers is 97 per cent efficient and comparable in effectiveness to a medical mask. The point to remember is that a facemask does not have to be 100 per cent efficient in blocking virus-laden particles to be useful, because obviously one with *some* efficiency is better than no facemask.

Will wearing a facemask reduce the severity of COVID-19 if someone is indeed infected even after wearing one? At the time of writing it was not clear.[11] What facemasks certainly do is limit exposure to the number of viruses to prevent infection altogether.

A homemade cloth facemask can be remarkably effective for blocking particles that might contain SARS-CoV-2.[12] Effective facemasks combine both mechanical and electrostatic filtering. Fabrics with very tight weaves, such as cotton with high thread counts, are preferable as a mechanical barrier. Chiffon, natural silk and flannel can be used as an internal, second layer for electrostatic filtering. By combining layers for a hybrid mask, at least 80 per cent of particles smaller than 300 nanometres and more than 90 per cent of particles larger than 300 nanometres can be filtered out.

How a facemask is worn is as important as what it is made from. For facemasks to work they must fit tightly over the nose and mouth, and not hang loosely under the nose. Having a thick beard can prevent the formation of a tight seal, and special respirators that account for beards kept for religious or personal reasons have been created. Facemasks with see-through sections near the mouth have also been created for those who are hearing-impaired. Surgical masks need to be pinched near the nose before use. Foggy eyewear is a sign that exhaled air is being forced up to the eyes. A small adhesive bandage applied on the mask near the nose can create a better seal. N95 masks can filter out 95 per cent of airborne particles, but there must be no loose pockets of air.

The wearer should wash hands with soap and water before wearing a facemask. The facemask should be secured without touching the face, ensuring there is a tight fit. When the facemask is removed, it should also be done without touching the face, and the user should promptly wash hands with soap and water.

Cloth facemasks should be washed in soap and warm water. Repeated washing will stretch natural fabric yarns over time, reducing filtration efficiency. Facemasks can be decontaminated for up to ten cycles without losing their filtration efficiency, but then materials start to degrade and loosen. N95 masks can be reused after decontamination in ultraviolet light.

At the time of writing, there were no large controlled studies of the check on transmission of SARS-CoV-2 in people wearing homemade facemasks daily. There is still scant evidence regarding capture of small aerosolized particles that might be exhaled, especially by people who are not showing symptoms but are infectious. The evidence is mostly indirect.

Studies of the physical properties of different materials and their effectiveness in capturing particles in laboratory environments have guided policy on the use of facemasks. In one particular experiment using sensitive light-scattering, a damp homemade cloth facemask reduced the droplets that were emitted while speaking.

Inferences based on the trajectories in countries where facemasks are prevalent compared to countries where they're not have also steered discussions. Facemasks were routinely used in Taiwan, Hong Kong, mainland China, Singapore and South Korea to slow the spread of respiratory illnesses even before the pandemic struck. During the pandemic, these countries were hit early, but proceeded on a slower trajectory than other countries which did not embrace masks early and willingly.

To ensure that facemasks are worn in public many countries such as Germany and Singapore instituted fines for non-compliance. Unfortunately, in many other countries, such as the United States, wearing a facemask became an ideological issue instead of a matter in the realm of public healthcare. The point that should have been reinforced was that wearing a facemask was not simply a measure to protect the wearer, but to protect others *from* the wearer—and as such, both a personal and a community measure to stop the spread of a highly infectious disease.

If facemasks work, why do we need social distancing? And if social distancing works, why do we need lockdowns? The reason is simple. It's all a matter of doing a proper risk assessment and analysing suitable trade-offs. We want to layer as many measures as we can to reduce risk.

At one end of the spectrum is imposing lockdowns which slow the spread of SARS-CoV-2 superbly when implemented fully for an adequate amount of time, but come at great social, psychological and economic costs. At the other end of the spectrum is doing nothing and succumbing to wishful thinking—hoping the disease is not as detrimental as envisaged, environmental heat and humidity kick in and slow the spread of the virus below a threshold, and innate immunity protects the population. Somewhere between these opposing extremes are measures that can be implemented relatively easily and universally such as the wearing of facemasks.

Social distancing alone may be inadequate in slowing down the spread of the virus, because there's a good chance of the virus sticking in the air longer, and for greater distances in aerosols, in crowded spaces indoors. And as we've just established, masks haven't been demonstrated to reduce the chance of spread completely.

Much of the initial reticence in advising the public to wear facemasks stemmed from a concern that there would be a scarcity of personal protective equipment for healthcare professionals at the start of the pandemic. In February 2020, the US Surgeon General tweeted that masks were 'NOT effective in preventing general public' from getting infected and that buying facemasks may put healthcare workers at risk.[13] This statement created unnecessary confusion by hinting that facemasks only stop spread for certain people, but not for others, which was not true. It also missed an obvious point that the general public need not use personal protective equipment, which may be scarce during a pandemic. Later, guidance was provided on the construction of cloth facemasks, and on how to use them.

Another criticism of facemasks was that they somehow lulled the wearer into a sense of complacency. While this assumption is theoretically possible, is it based on any actual data? There is little evidence of compensatory risky behaviour at the individual level, and the upside of wearing facemasks is far greater. Seatbelts and helmets do not lead to more risky driving.

Instead, it can be argued that there is an advantage to ensuring that facemasks are worn universally. Seeing other people wear facemasks is a normative reminder for responsible practices as well as measures such as handwashing, reduced face-touching and physical distancing. A computer scientist measured over 12,000 interactions between people in masked and unmasked situations and found that wearing a facemask correlated to passers-by walking at a greater distance from one another.[14] Simply viewing facemasks reminded people of other social-distancing practices.

## How stable is the coronavirus?

During an infectious period, an undiagnosed infectious person might contaminate surfaces and objects between ten and hundred times. From the buttons inside lifts to smartphones, there are so many touch-activated devices that our hands can pick up virus particles from and pass on.

To understand what our chances are of getting sick, we need to know how much virus is needed to cause an infection. This is known as the infectious dose and it is usually described as the number of pathogens that can infect half of a susceptible population. A virus with a low infectious dose is likely to be very contagious in populations that are susceptible to infection.

Right now, the infectious dose for SARS-CoV-2 isn't known. Testing transmission in animals that can get infected helps answer this question, even if animals are not perfect proxies for human infections.

For SARS coronavirus, it has been calculated that if a group of people are exposed to 280 virus particles each, around half will get infected. This is in the range for other coronaviruses that cause common cold and influenza. For now, there's no reason to suspect that SARS-CoV-2 will be different from all these other viruses.

On the other hand, infection with tuberculosis can happen after inhaling only ten bacteria.

We are all very interested in knowing what our chances of infection are from surfaces and from everyday objects like books packages, groceries and clothes. Overall, the risk is very low.[15] A number of things have to happen for spread of the virus from surfaces or objects. Collectively, these steps reduce risk.

First, someone who is infected has to contaminate a surface by coughing, sneezing, or touching it with infected hands. Then, the virus has to remain at a viable concentration in specific conditions of light, humidity and temperature. From the moment the surface is infected, the amount of virus on it decreases over time. The decay of the amount of virus has been shown to be very rapid. For example, half of SARS-CoV-2 particles applied to paper or cloth decay in thirty minutes.

Most importantly, it isn't enough for a surface to be contaminated. SARS-CoV-2 has to get inside a person's body. For this to occur, the infected surface with viable virus has to be touched and the virus has to enter by subsequent contamination of the nose, eyes, or mouth.

The role of disinfection in controlling the spread of disease is well-documented. Railway carriages were disinfected regularly during a plague outbreak in India in 1897, the same year of the Epidemic Disease Act. Disinfection works by greatly reducing the number of viable infectious agents over time. They do not work instantaneously. A disinfectant should completely wet a potentially contaminated surface. It should also be allowed to sit on a surface for a few minutes before being wiped off. Using a spray and immediately wiping does not fulfil these criteria and may not be adequate for disinfection.

Fortunately, unlike some other viruses that have a tough protein capsid, enveloped viruses like SARS-CoV-2 which have a lipid coating can be easily inactivated.[16] Ethyl alcohol, Isopropyl alcohol, bleach, hydrogen peroxide, citric acid and quaternary ammonium salts can break down the virus and render it harmless. Soap works very well for hands. For clothes, washing in warm water is recommended.

Proper handwashing should be done for twenty seconds. A good lather should cover all parts of the hands. Most of the data on handwashing is from other viruses such as SARS and influenza. Handwashing certainly reduces transmission in children as expected.

According to the US FDA there is 'no evidence of food packaging being associated with the transmission of the coronavirus. However, if you wish, you can wipe down product packaging and allow it to air dry, as an extra precaution'.[17]

Fruits and vegetables should be rinsed with clean water. Washing vegetables and fruits with soap can cause illness due to the ingestion of residues and has been discouraged by multiple organizations including the US Department of Agriculture: this is potentially harmful and should be avoided.

A general rule of thumb is that in lower temperatures, more virus particles are stable for longer. At temperatures inside a refrigerator, viruses may remain viable for weeks. While at room temperature, it is so for a much shorter time. Ramping temperatures up accelerates the process of degradation. In an experiment, at 56°C, thirty minutes was enough to get rid of most of the virus, while at 70°C, it only took five minutes.

SARS-CoV-2 persists for a longer period on hard surfaces like doorknobs and lift buttons, compared to soft ones like articles of clothing. For SARS, the WHO recommended cleaning high-touch surfaces every two hours. Given the similar surface stability of SARS-CoV-2, this was thought to be an acceptable approach. However, experts have stated that 'we are overcleaning in response to COVID-19' because even by December 2020 there weren't clear indications of transmission from surfaces.[18]

SARS-CoV-2 had been detected for up to four hours on copper, up to a day on cardboard and up to two to three days on plastic and stainless steel.[19] Another study found that SARS-CoV-2 could not be detected on paper after three hours, on cloth after two days and on stainless steel after seven days. It is important to keep in mind that the amount of virus drops very quickly.[20] Even on stainless steel, half of all virus particles could not be detected after six hours.

Scientists also test for viable virus in the natural environment after an outbreak. They can take samples where infections have occurred to check for virus.

In March 2020, 10 per cent of samples collected from the *Diamond Princess* cruise ship, where there was a major outbreak, tested positive for viral RNA.[21] These samples had been collected after cabins had been vacated, but before disinfection. In another study, 80 per cent of air and surface samples from rooms inside the University of Nebraska Medical Center in the US where infected patients stayed tested positive for virus.

It is careful to note how viability of a virus is determined.[22] Many tests of stability rely on RT-PCR, which isn't the same as finding infectious virus. We still need to establish a direct link between various surfaces infected with viruses and actual infections.

Overall, the data through 2020 indicated that the risk of infection from surfaces was highest immediately after the surface had been contaminated by someone who was infectious, and overall, minuscule.

## Infections mainly occur indoors

It is estimated that nine out of ten infections happen indoors with people in close quarters in face-to-face situations. This makes it apparent that proper implementation of measures to avoid crowded areas and close interactions with people in closed spaces indoors is key to preventing large outbreaks. Most people acquire an infection outside the home and will infect others in their own households. This has remained a consistent trend from early in the outbreak in Wuhan through to the end of 2020. Prevention of spread among family members by home isolation of those who are infected is difficult, if not impossible, because by the time the person who brought the infection home gets sick, he or she might've spread it to others. Use of common cooking vessels, plates, cups and cooking utensils, plus proximity makes it difficult to prevent infection in close quarters. Limited ventilation might also increase the chance of spread.

People in industrialized nations spend most of their time indoors, regardless of season. The spread of respiratory infections in indoor environments has been studied extensively. Therefore, it is imperative to ensure that the spread of the virus can be prevented while indoors as much as possible. In the presence of others who are not part of the same household and have unknown infection status, it is advisable to wear facemasks and maintain distance.

It is well established that casual interactions between people in well-ventilated places under conditions of social distancing limit the risk of infection. You are unlikely to get infected from going on a walk, run or bike-ride in the middle of the day: a combination of air, light and temperature lowers the chance. Even if you can't always maintain appropriate social distancing, you will have very transient interactions in an environment that is not conducive to viral spread.

Physically separating people from one another is an effective way to prevent infection. In hospitals this can be achieved through specialized wards for COVID-19 patients with negative pressure chambers (isolation rooms). High-efficiency particulate air (HEPA) filters can trap 300 nanometre particles with greater than 99.9 per cent efficiency, making them suitable, though expensive, for regular use.

Temperature and humidity inactivate viruses by impacting the viral lipid membrane. Lower temperature promotes stability of influenza viruses. To prevent spread, humidifying air to about

40-60 per cent has been suggested especially in the colder, drier months of the year. Wearing face covering not only keeps the nose and mouth germ-free, it also keeps them warm and moist. Open spaces with ventilation are less conducive to the spread of viruses.

Crowds should also be avoided. Another measure is increasing the airflow and preventing recirculation of air that might be laden with aerosols containing virus particles. HEPA filtration and purifier systems also work in removing most droplets and aerosols containing SARS-CoV-2. All these measures, along with disinfection, can reduce risk of infections indoors.

In addition to facemasks, eye protection has been shown to decrease the likelihood of infection through the eyes. SARS-CoV-2 particles can invade the conjunctiva from where it can proceed to the respiratory system. However, virus particles do not have a simple path to the respiratory system from the eyes and this is, at best, a secondary route of infection.

Airplanes pose unique challenges because they represent confined spaces. Transmission of SARS-CoV-2 on airplanes has been reported.[23] Flights are typically of reasonably long durations, air is recirculated and there are numerous surfaces that must be touched. Airplanes have HEPA filters that remove virus-laden aerosols and droplets, but the interior environment is still prone to transmission. Many planes kept middle seats unoccupied and have been sanitizing before and after flights: the impact of these steps have not been tested adequately. Simple steps to minimize the chance of infection include using the washroom before boarding, avoiding moving around on the plane as much as possible, requesting a window seat (since it is most isolated), sanitizing surfaces, avoiding meals and wearing a mask and a face-shield before, during and after a flight.

Overall, much was known by the end of 2020 regarding the relative risk of transmission compared to when the pandemic started. Some of the factors are summarized in the table below.

Relative risk of SARS-CoV-2 transmission

| Factors | Lowest risk | Highest risk |
|---|---|---|
| *Environmental factors* | | |
| Proximity | Interactions >2m | Interactions <1m |
| Duration | Less than a few minutes | Several hours |
| Density | Spread out | Crowded in small spaces |
| Location | Outdoors or well-ventilated indoors | Poorly ventilated indoors |
| Environmental conditions | Normal indoor temperature, humidity and fresh air | Low temperature, low humidity |
| Viral emission | Passive activities, face coverings | Singing, loud talking, no face coverings |
| Shared surfaces | Good cleaning, rarely touched areas | Infrequent cleaning, high-touch areas |
| *Human factors* | | |
| Frequency of contact | Infrequent contact, positive cases isolated | Daily regular contact |
| Hygiene | Proper hand hygiene, face coverings | Poor hand hygiene, no face coverings |
| Networks | Small bubble of contacts | Shared space with strangers |
| Occupation | Limited dealings with the public | Public-facing, healthcare sector, and/or long working hours |
| Socioeconomic factors | Work from home, ability to isolate | Poverty, inability to isolate, crowded housing |

*Source:* Modified from 'SARS-CoV-2: Transmission Routes and Environments, UK Government Office of Science'[24]

# 13

# Spread

Pandemics are like snowflakes: no two are exactly alike. But we can still categorize how severe a pandemic is based on three factors. A pandemic signifies global spread, so the factor that probably comes to mind first is how infectious a disease is. But the prime element that dictates just how serious a pandemic gets is the number of deaths it causes. These two numbers alone don't dictate the severity of the pandemic. We also need to look at how the disease progresses and when it is transmitted. A disease that can be spread easily through the airborne route is different from one that can be spread by a water route.

There are four factors that determine the progression of an infectious disease such as COVID-19.[1] First, and foremost, is obviously the infectious agent, in this case, the virus. Everything starts from the minuscule infectious particle with a simple set of genes. Then, there's the transmission process. There's no spread unless there's an efficient process by which the virus can be spread. The third link is the host. This is where the virus will multiply. An infection might result in a disease with no symptoms whatsoever to severe deterioration to the point of death. COVID-19 spans the entire range. By human-to-human transmission, the host also provides a way for the virus to spread. The fourth chain of infection is the environment—population density, temperature and air pollution are all factors in the transmission of a respiratory disease.

The interplay of all these factors plays out at the population level. The decision on how best to protect a population must be made with as much information as possible, but during a pandemic not all the information will be available or accurate.

In addition, there are complex ethical, social, economic, educational and health issues at play in determining what kinds of measures need to be taken. Is a lockdown necessary? And if so when is the best time to apply one? What is the best way to lift one? And these measures must be evaluated in real-time and in comparison to local data, human needs and incoming information from other countries on what works best.

## Why the world stopped for COVID-19

COVID-19 is unlike any other disease we have seen in our lives.

- COVID-19 can spread through people who are infected but are not yet sick, those who have mild symptoms which they will not get checked up, and those who will never get sick. Identifying and isolating are huge problems because many have silent infections.
- COVID-19 is primarily a respiratory infectious disease (though there are other complications). Respiratory infectious diseases pose major challenges compared to other types of infectious diseases. Breathing is not optional.
- Transmission of COVID-19 occurs very easily. Unchecked, each person may infect an average of more than two uninfected people. To slow the spread of an infectious disease in a population that has little immunity to it, this number must go down to less than one.
- COVID-19 is lethal. If unchecked, vulnerable populations such as the elderly and those with heart disease and other conditions

will die in large numbers. In addition, many times more people will get very sick. COVID-19 is not like coronaviruses that are common in humans, and that that cause the common cold. COVID-19 is not like the influenza subtype H1N1 that caused the last pandemic in 2009, which was probably less fatal than seasonal influenza. This is a serious disease.

To summarize, a disease can be much more lethal than COVID-19 but be limited in the manner in which it spreads and how fast it spreads. A disease can be much more contagious than COVID-19 and spread faster but be very mild and not cause major sickness or death in a substantial portion of the population.

## Outbreaks, epidemics and pandemics

We need to know a few terms about how diseases are spread. An *endemic* disease is one that exists in people at a low level. An endemic disease is an established disease that isn't going away. The human coronaviruses that circulate in people and cause common colds are endemic. Flu subtypes that cause annual or seasonal flu are also endemic. A newly emerged disease can end up vanishing, being eradicated, posing a low-level, persistent threat, or becoming endemic. Most experts think SARS-CoV-2 will become an endemic disease once the pandemic ends.

A rapid increase in cases of an infectious disease is called an *epidemic*. The SARS outbreak became an epidemic. HIV/AIDS spread much more slowly but is considered an epidemic (and one that is ongoing in certain parts of the world).

An epidemic starts out as an outbreak, which is a loosely associated set of cases. There's no clear definition of what constitutes an outbreak. MERS is sporadic and has fortunately not graduated from an outbreak to an epidemic. COVID-19 was initially identified as an outbreak in Wuhan when cases of pneumonia of an unknown cause were identified.

There's no formal definition of a *pandemic*, but the WHO decides that when an epidemic has spread over a few continents rapidly, it's a pandemic. A pandemic in the modern era typically occurs for a new disease for which people don't have much immunity. COVID-19 is the first pandemic caused by a coronavirus. Using a very narrow definition we can say that a pandemic is the sudden and rapid occurrence of an infectious disease that spreads easily and impacts many places globally. Before the existence of the WHO, there were no formal definitions of pandemics, and even today there's a bit of grey area as to what constitutes a pandemic. In the nineteenth century several cholera pandemics arose in India. The twentieth century is mainly known for devastating influenza pandemics.

After the WHO declared the 2009 H1N1 influenza outbreak a pandemic, there was controversy since it did not cause severe illness in large swathes of the world as had been initially feared. The WHO clarified that disease severity is not a criterion for declaring a pandemic.

How are outbreaks, epidemics and pandemics related? Some outbreaks lead to epidemics, and only a few epidemics (fortunately for us) lead to pandemics.

Now let's review how cases are grouped together.

*A cluster of infections* occurs at the same time in the same area. Clusters are often linked by transmission. They may or may not be traced to a specific event. Identification of a cluster is a good trigger that something needs to be done in the affected area to stop further spread. *Community transmission* is the spread of an infectious disease among people in an area without travel history, linking infections or contact with a confirmed case. There's no clear explanation for how these infections are being transmitted.

It is worth pointing out that identifying whether an area is experiencing a defined cluster of infections or community transmission helps to determine what measures need to be taken to control further spread of the virus. They do not indicate that the virus has altered biologically in any way or that the severity of the disease has changed. With SARS-CoV-2 spread, the virus can cause cluster infections in one place, and may have already passed on to broader community transmission in another.

The *incubation period* is the time between when someone gets infected and when he or she notices symptoms of COVID-19. Estimates of the incubation period for COVID-19 range from two to fourteen days, with an average of around five to six days.

## Silent infections

On 8 June 2020, a WHO official raised a storm with a comment that silent spread of SARS-CoV-2 is infrequent. The technical lead for the WHO coronavirus response said, 'From the data we have, it still seems to be rare that an asymptomatic person actually transmits onward to a secondary individual.'[2]

The following day, the WHO clarified that the statement was misunderstood and that scientists had not yet determined how often spread by those who had no symptoms was occurring.[3]

How much is asymptomatic spread of SARS-CoV-2 responsible for the rapid spread of the pandemic? One of the first studies indicated as many as 80 per cent of infections are asymptomatic or result in mild COVID-19. Approximately 14 per cent have severe disease, and 5-6 per cent are critically ill.[4]

The first known death from COVID-19 in Italy occurred on 21 February 2020 in Vò, a small town near Venice. Authorities in Italy had a strong reaction to the outbreak, and the entire municipality was put under lockdown for fourteen days, during which time nearly all 3200 residents were tested for the virus twice. Mass testing in conjunction with the lockdown was key to eliminating COVID-19 from the area. Since nearly everyone was tested, Vò gave us one of the first opportunities to get a sense of the extent of silent infections. Over 40 per cent of those who were infected in Vò ended up testing positive but being asymptomatic: they never got sick.[5]

Between 27 April and 11 May 2020, researchers in Spain tested over 61,000 people for antibodies to SARS-CoV-2 and found that one-third of them had no symptoms.[6] In total, around 5 per cent of those who were tested were positive. If extrapolated to the entire country that would mean that around one million people had silent infections.

The US CDC had also put together pandemic planning scenarios by 20 May that accounted for roughly one-quarter to half of all infections being asymptomatic.[7] A review of existing studies agreed with this assessment, estimating that asymptomatic people account for 40 per cent to 45 per cent of SARS-CoV-2 infections, and that they transmit the virus to others for an extended period, perhaps longer than fourteen days.[8] India's own ICMR commented in April that around 80 per cent of cases were asymptomatic but didn't parse out those who later develop symptoms.[9] In October, an analysis that combined data from thirteen studies involving over 21,000 people concluded that around 17 per cent of people were asymptomatic.[10]

Why has there been so much disparity in dealing with these numbers?

First, it is important to note that we don't typically consider infections without clinical disease, or in other words a scenario in which not everyone who is infected feels sick.

Asymptomatic infections for many viral infections can be detected from isolating the virus or testing for it either through an RT-PCR or antigen or antibody tests. It's a laborious process and normally in our day-to-day lives we don't think about it at all. That's because, even the symptomatic form of many infections is mild and self-limiting. When the rest of our families are down with the flu, but we are not, we don't entertain the possibility that we might be harbouring asymptomatic infections. Instead, we always assume that we weren't infected in the first place.

Even people who do get sick with COVID-19 go through a phase of one or two days just before symptoms start to show up when they can spread the virus without knowing it.[11] The time before someone is sick is the *pre-symptomatic phase* and unfortunately this is also quite infectious. In those who get sick, the virus is most transmissible just before and around the time symptoms start to show up. It's believed that around half of transmission in those who end up with symptomatic COVID-19 happens during the pre-symptomatic phase.

If matters weren't complicated enough, there's a third group of people who may have very mild symptoms: in such *paucisymptomatic*, or mild cases, sufferers may shrug off the symptoms or associate them with other illnesses such as the common cold or a slight flu. Paucisymptomatic individuals sometimes have atypical infections: they may have only one symptom out of many, or uncommon symptoms that don't fit the profile of the disease.

It's also natural to wonder how those with asymptomatic infections spread the virus. They themselves may be unaware they're infected. In the stages of greatest infectiousness, simply breathing and talking can spread viruses. Talking louder or singing will release even more particles. And while the actual viral load of someone who is talking loudly might be lower than someone who is sneezing large droplets, over a long time the cumulative infectious dose that someone who is not infected gets does add up.

Why should we worry about silent infections? If asymptomatic people didn't have any capacity to spread the virus, these infections would reach dead-ends and we wouldn't bother as much. The problem is that asymptomatic people can go on with their normal lives, all the while spreading the virus, whereas sick people are more likely to either be identified and be isolated because of their symptoms or stay at home. Asymptomatic spread poses a huge challenge to controlling disease and is one of the defining hallmarks of SARS-CoV-2 compared to other recently emerged coronaviruses that cause SARS and MERS.

The CDC certainly seems to think that the infectiousness of an asymptomatic individual is anywhere from half to equal to that of a person who is symptomatic and sick.[12] While subsequent studies have had wildly different numbers for asymptomatic spread, symptom-based control has not been able to control the disease, unlike in the case of SARS.

The presence of many asymptomatic individuals will decrease the infection fatality rate by increasing the denominator of those who are infected but not dying. This means that a country might also approach herd immunity faster.

On the flipside, apart from the major difficulty in controlling spread, it also makes tracing contacts harder. If a fever is not a reliable and consistent indicator of infection with SARS-CoV-2, having a temperature gun may look good as 'security theatre', but have only a negligible effect in controlling disease. A good tenet to evade silent spread is to consider everyone potentially infected (including yourself) if you are in an area where there is an outbreak, so that you can prevent both inward and outward transmission.

The traits of a pandemic strain of influenza appear only after its emergence, but we do know a lot about the asymptomatic and pre-symptomatic spread of influenza. Most people infected with influenza virus develop symptomatic illness (with fever and sore throat or cough), but as many as one-third to half of those who are infected might have asymptomatic or paucisymptomatic infections.[13] Seasonal strains of influenza also typically have about one to two days of pre-symptomatic infectiousness. So, the entire spectrum from no symptoms to mild symptoms to severe disease is also observed in influenza.

Why might SARS-CoV-2 have asymptomatic and pre-symptomatic spread when the related SARS coronavirus did not? Knowing this is key to understanding the difference in spread between the two diseases and why one became a pandemic and the other did not. Early on in infection, SARS-CoV-2 is a disease of the upper respiratory tract (nose and throat) and at that time the symptoms are mild or non-existent. This distinguishes it from SARS coronavirus which replicated primarily in the lower respiratory tract. Under 10 per cent of those who were infected with SARS and MERS might've had asymptomatic infections, but they probably were not able to transmit the disease to others efficiently.

A final tantalizing question relates to why some people harbour silent infections at all while others who (on paper, at least) have similar risk factors develop serious COVID-19? Several theories have been postulated. There are likely genetic components to susceptibility. But recent studies have also indicated that earlier exposure to human coronaviruses trigger immune responses, and immune memory with T-cells can limit serious infection.[14] Or in other words, not everyone is equally susceptible to infection. These are all excellent lines of inquiry that will require further study.

# 14

# Curve

An epidemic curve is a visual representation of newly occurring reported cases over time. Measures are used to slow down the growth in daily cases to reduce the peak (the height of the curve), total cases (the area in the curve) and the burden on the healthcare system. By shifting the curve to the right, we delay the peak so that we buy more time. This provides healthcare professionals the opportunity to learn more about the disease and how to treat it. It allows existing repurposed drugs to be tested and scaled up. And it provides vital months for new drugs and vaccines to go into clinical trials, be mass produced, and administered to populations. 'Flattening the curve' allows us to learn and to adapt.

When we look at the daily new cases that have been identified and reported over time, they will reach a peak. Depending on the measures that are taken and their effectiveness, the peak might be taller or shorter. Of course, when we think of a peak, we may expect to see a well-defined feature such Mt Everest. But what we may observe is a plateau like the Deccan Plateau much in the manner that the epidemic peak of new cases was for the United States from mid-April through June. This is simply because for large, heterogeneous countries like India, the US and Brazil, the country-curve is the sum of many different places at different points in their respective epidemic curves. What we will also be

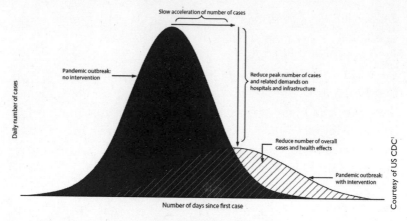

Flattening the curve

looking at are different curves for smaller regions because control measures in Mumbai will be different from those in Kerala, and those in Chhattisgarh will be different from those on the Andaman Islands (even though all are part of India). Containment zones are set up to identify and contain infections in regions that are severely affected.

The epidemic curve transformed from a series of visual representations for disease spread in the nineteenth century to tools for prediction in the early twentieth century and then to a set of proactive gears for determining the effectiveness of measures in the twenty-first.[2] During the COVID-19 pandemic, everyone got a crash course in epidemiology. For some, looking at new cases and deaths by city, state and country became a daily ritual. Data was available to anyone with access to the Internet, something which may not have been available in pandemics in prior centuries.

The terms 'flattening the curve' and 'herd immunity' became a part of common parlance. Many of us took a keen interest in measures to slow the spread of the virus and flatten the peak of the epidemic curve. Where did 'flattening the curve' as an individual and collective responsibility come from? It came from a very influential influenza pandemic preparedness plan.

In 2007 the US CDC drafted a plan to guide strategies in the event of an influenza pandemic. The plan was astute in predicting that hospitals would be overrun in an unmitigated pandemic. At that time, the best analyses on how social-distancing measures had been implemented and countered mortalities in US cities were available for the H1N1 pandemic of 1918: cities that implemented measures early fared better.[3] The CDC noted the effects, and predicting that another influenza pandemic was inevitable, recommended implementing measures to buy time and decrease the adverse impacts of a peak. 'Flattening the curve' was born. After the 2009 H1N1 influenza pandemic, this document was superseded by a revision, which also makes a riveting read.[4]

Measures that flatten the curve don't cure the disease or increase immunity. Or in other words, once a measure is removed, the threat of infection may re-emerge.

Prior to the coronavirus pandemic, the pandemics that were most similar in size and scope were associated with newly emergent subtypes of influenza. Measures such as personal hygiene (handwashing, throwing away used tissue paper), physical distancing, closing schools and wearing facemasks were implemented in past influenza pandemics and are measures that have been around for more than a century. Much of the data on the effectiveness of school and workplace closures stem from the H1N1 influenza pandemic of 1918.

Among all viruses that have infected humans, SARS-CoV-2 is most like the SARS coronavirus virologically. But SARS was controlled before becoming a devastating pandemic. This was possible because SARS was not spread significantly by those who were not sick. Peak infectiousness happened days *after* symptoms showed up, so patients could be isolated successfully. There were a few superspreaders and superspreading events and healthcare workers were disproportionately infected, but by the summer of 2003, infections were completely under control.

SARS-CoV-2 is the first pandemic in the modern era caused by a coronavirus. Influenza viruses have caused many pandemics, and much of what we know about controlling transmission, modelling epidemics and managing respiratory diseases comes from influenza pandemics. From the perspective of epidemiology, SARS-CoV-2 resembles influenza viruses in many ways.

The challenges of controlling influenza viruses apply to controlling SARS-CoV-2. Notably, influenza is also known to spread through 'silent infections' from those who are asymptomatic and don't feel sick. We tend to think of fever as emblematic of flu, but many influenza infections are not accompanied by fever. Silent spread can also happen in pre-symptomatic cases of influenza. For example, for the 2009 H1N1 influenza pandemic, some people who got sick were infectious a day before symptoms showed up.

Both are viruses with RNA as genetic material, of approximately similar size, and have a lipid enveloped layer. Both are relatively delicate viruses and that's why handwashing and chemical inactivation concepts are broadly applicable. Transmission is by respiratory droplet, aerosols and on surfaces, though there are notable differences in properties of different influenza and coronaviruses. Steps to control the transmission of SARS-CoV-2 resulted in shortening of the season for recurring influenza in the northern hemisphere.[5]

How much influenza virus someone has in their upper respiratory tract determines how easily they spread the virus. This is similar to COVID-19. Many of the symptoms of the flu and COVID-19 are non-specific to the disease, making it difficult to know what we have—someone can have a fever and cough with either disease.

Just as underlying conditions can make things worse for those suffering from COVID-19, they can do the same for those suffering from influenza: those who have lung disease, bronchitis, heart conditions and emphysema can suffer from more serious flu. (But COVID-19 does not always have the same symptoms as the flu either, because it shows up in many different organs apart from the lungs. The seasonal flu is still mainly a respiratory disease.)

Both for influenza pandemics and for the COVID-19 pandemic, studies have shown that the timing of measures is critical. Reacting to a dire situation on the ground is less effective than proactively trying to anticipate it. A paradigm for dealing with a pandemic that has the potential for mass fatalities is that it is better to overreact than to underreact.

There are differences between influenza and coronaviruses, of course. The genetic material of influenza viruses is broken into pieces. Influenza viruses mutate at a faster rate than coronaviruses because they make sloppier copies of their genetic material. The receptors (and consequently some of the cells that can be infected) are different.

Influenza cycles through faster. Pandemic influenza is hard to control compared to COVID-19 because the incubation period is around two days (compared to five to six days for COVID-19). COVID-19 at least gives us time to contact trace and isolate patients. For most influenza, one person usually infects less than two other people on average which is less than the average for SARS-CoV-2 (the exception was the H1N1 subtype which started the pandemic in 1918 which may have been as infectious as SARS-CoV-2).

But cases of influenza can double in about three days, making exponential spread rapid and increase by ten times in one or two weeks. Influenza might cycle through in six weeks and might need three months for public health measures. It became clear in 2020 that SARS-CoV-2 has a longer lag time and disease cycle.

SARS-CoV-2 is probably in the order of ten to twenty times more lethal than seasonal influenza. Based on what we know, SARS-CoV-2 is more severe than recent influenza pandemics and has the potential to be a little less severe than the H1N1 influenza pandemic of 1918: without preventative measures, the pandemic had the potential to cause millions of deaths in India alone.

Closing schools is a highly effective measure for the control of influenza because children transmit and get infections easily. Based on what we know, small children are less likely to get infected with SARS-CoV-2. Further, by December it became clear that while children can get infected, if preventative measures are taken, they are less likely to get infected at school than they are at home and other places.

SARS-CoV-2 appears to be more transmissible than most influenza seasonal and pandemic influenza viruses. In terms of deaths, by the time the pandemic ends, COVID-19 will be worse than the influenza pandemics of 1957, 1968 and 2009.

Modern medicine and technology, better surveillance, molecular detection of viruses and quicker responses almost certainly guarantee that the COVID-19 pandemic won't be as catastrophically fatal as the 1918 H1N1 influenza pandemic.

## The patient is the community

Infectious disease epidemiologists study how often infectious diseases occur in different people and how they spread. The US CDC puts the difference between an epidemiologist who is a public health official and a doctor, whom you and I might see when we're sick, quite aptly : 'The clinician is concerned about the health of an individual; the epidemiologist is concerned about the collective health of the people in a community or population. In other words, the clinician's "patient" is the individual; the epidemiologist's "patient" is the community.'[6]

Epidemiologists assess the effects of public health measures on disease control. Preventative measures that don't involve a vaccine or a drug are often the only approaches available to slow or stop the spread of a disease at the start of an epidemic. They're also referred to as non-pharmaceutical interventions. They can be categorized into community-level approaches that require some level of coordination and individual measures that people take themselves. In addition, there are also environmental measures such as the use of disinfectants that may be applied for the duration of an outbreak. The two goals of measures are to prevent people from getting sick and to save lives: this is achieved by reducing transmission.

How well a virus transmits in a new population depends on how well it is adapted for transmission in the host. These are biological factors internal to the virus and to the host. There are also external factors related to the environment including the patterns of spread. To understand transmission all of these must be considered in real-time as new information becomes available.

For a respiratory infectious disease, the success of all measures hinges on the ability to reduce contact between those who are infected and those who are not. As such, it requires identifying those who are infected through testing, those who are susceptible, and those who are immune. It also involves increasing the distance between people and reducing the number of contacts.

The stark reality is that early decisions on how to protect the public during the COVID-19 pandemic had to be made in the 'fog of war', in the midst of uncertainty around modes of transmission, extent of infectivity and true fatality rates. (A similar scenario on a smaller scale played out in the UK in December with the discovery of a new variant with possibly enhanced transmission). In addition, prior to the current pandemic there were few studies on the effectiveness of various preventative measures. What little information we had was mainly from the relatively mild 2009 H1N1 influenza pandemic and studies that looked back at the 1918 H1N1 influenza pandemic.

## Understanding the numbers

It truly is a wonderful time to be alive to be able to see data as it comes in and to at least feel that we can change the trajectory of the epidemic curve. But paradoxically, the superabundance of information readily available to anyone with Internet access also leads to a sense of helplessness because we cannot push the daily or weekly numbers in the downward direction. The most we can personally do is to take measures—wear masks, physically distance ourselves from others, avoid crowds, maintain hand hygiene.

During a pandemic, it is possible to get caught up in numbers presented without a clear explanation of why they are important and what they mean. Here are the five metrics that are useful to understanding what is going on. Each presents caveats but, taken together, they offer a reasonable snapshot of trends:[7]

*Confirmed new cases:* Confirmed numbers of cases are presented daily. If no one is tested, there are no new cases, but of course that doesn't mean infections magically vanish. Conversely, if everyone is tested, numbers are accurate, but this is not a practical solution. There is a middle ground between testing everyone and testing no one. During an active outbreak, the proportion of positive results may decrease as more tests are performed.

The highest priority for testing should be reserved for those who are symptomatic—especially hospitalized patients, vulnerable residents in long-term healthcare settings, migrant shelters and jails, and essential workers in high-risk situations. People without symptoms also need to be tested, especially if they have a high chance of being exposed to those who have tested positive. Combined with contact tracing, testing is a demonstrably effective measure. Beyond these conditions, clinicians will follow appropriate guidelines at the time with the understanding that test reagents, time and facilities are an exhaustible resource.

Reported daily numbers are subject to persistent errors, and moving averages tend to smooth fluctuations due to underreporting artifacts (sometimes for a reason as mundane as fewer tests run on weekends). Confirmed new cases are a subset of all cases because of underreporting and silent infections (both asymptomatic and pre-symptomatic) and lack of testing.

*Confirmed deaths attributed to COVID-19:* Deaths lag infections and confirmed cases by a few weeks, but this is a crucial metric that can be used to estimate the number of *actual* deaths, which will be more than reported deaths under most practical circumstances. Confirmed deaths are underreported because not all COVID-19 deaths can be identified. Many deaths due to a COVID-19 associated underlying condition will list that condition as the cause of death instead of COVID-19. A confirmed COVID-19 death also requires a prior diagnostic test to have yielded a positive.

*Excess mortality:* While confirmed deaths are an underrepresentation, excess mortality is an overrepresentation because the cause of death is unspecified. Any spike in 'pneumonia-like illness' in a region in a time period must be examined. But tests are not available everywhere and excess deaths due to pneumonia-like illness over comparable time periods is concerning. During the pandemic many of these excess deaths are due to COVID-19.

*Hospital capacity:* This metric can be looked at both as capacity of ICU beds and percentage of capacity that is occupied. These are exceptionally useful to assess the acute burden on a healthcare system. Visits to emergency rooms are also a metric that can be tracked.

*Prevalence:* This metric is useful to identify how many people in a population have already been infected. It relies on accurate detection of antibodies in the blood of donors. Antibodies can take weeks to rise to detectable levels in symptomatic cases, and thus have a more limited utility in diagnosing and stopping spread during the early phase of infection. Antibody tests may not also tell us if a person is immune to SARS-CoV-2 infection. This is both due to limitations on the accuracy of these tests and in our knowledge of how many and what kind of antibodies are needed for protection. The problem with antibody tests is that false positives can artificially inflate the proportion of the population that has antibodies. This is a particularly important issue when the true prevalence of a disease is low.

# 15

# Lethality

Central to how to react to the global spread of a new disease is the question: *just how deadly is it?*

We may assume that infection with SARS-CoV-2 results in a disease with a very high chance of fatality based on what we hear. News organizations report on the most serious cases that result in death. That is to be expected because they have a responsibility to inform. A harrowing personal account is important and newsworthy, but it is not necessarily representative of a population, and it may not contain information that can be used to come to full terms with an ongoing public health crisis.

On the other hand, that limitation equally applies to us when we share our own experiences of COVID-19. Some of us may have suffered through the disease and recovered after a protracted bout involving many potentially life-threatening symptoms. Or we may have been infected with no or relatively minor symptoms for just a few days. Each case represents one unique star in a galaxy of all possible outcomes. Each of these stars helps us to get a constellation of the disease in one moment in time to understand the lethality in a specific population.

Even though we know most people will recover from getting infected with SARS-CoV-2, it is a serious disease because of how lethal it is. At first pass, it may sound counterintuitive that we are worrying more about COVID-19 than we are about diseases that have much higher death rates, but we also must remember that it is highly transmissible. In terms of deaths, it is the worst pandemic in over a hundred years. In addition, a lot of people are very sick: fatality isn't a comprehensive metric.

It helps to visualize various levels of personal risk and prevalence in populations as concentric circles. The outermost, largest circle includes everyone who has been infected. Not everyone will get exposed to the virus, and even with the same exposure under precisely the same circumstances, not everyone will get infected. So, those who are infected represent only a fraction of the total population outside the circle. The next circle inside is the symptomatic disease, COVID-19: of those who are infected, a certain proportion of people, but not everyone, will get sick. This is a smaller circle. And within this circle, we can even imagine progressively smaller circles of increasingly serious conditions until we get to the smallest, which includes only people who die from the disease.

Now, I'd like to introduce the symptomatic *case fatality rate*. This is the proportion of people sick with a clinically defined disease who die. To calculate the case fatality rate, we take those who were sick as the denominator, and of those who were sick, the subset of people who die from the disease as the numerator. This fraction isn't greater than one and is usually represented as a percentage.

The case fatality rate is not the only number that we have to consider. There are also the people who were infected, who never got sick enough to have detectable symptoms of the disease. The *infection fatality rate* defines the portion of people who are infected who die. Because there will always be more infected people than sick people, the denominator for the infection fatality rate is greater than that for the case fatality rate.

The infection fatality rate is always lower than the case fatality rate for every disease because not everyone who is infected gets sick.

The infection fatality rate accounts for asymptomatic and undiagnosed infections, whereas the case fatality rate does not.

Let's imagine a completely new virus has popped up and has started to infect people all of a sudden. Everyone who gets infected shows a very visible symptom of disease: his or her skin turns green. Now, no other disease causes this condition so we can get a pretty clear diagnosis. No one has any immunity to this new virus and no one is infected without any symptoms. Some people, around 10 in 1000 people of those who get infected, get very sick and die, while the other 990 recover. Because of the very visible symptoms everyone who is infected gets detected. Because, in this case infection equates to disease, and there's limited variability in disease progressions, the case fatality rate of 1 per cent is easy to calculate.

Thinking about a made-up disease can help us to understand the main ways in which real infectious diseases are different: they follow no simple trajectories. And because they do not, grasping true fatality rates for a real disease like COVID-19 is difficult. It is extremely hard to get firm numbers of fatality, especially while a pandemic is ongoing. We do not know exactly how many people are infected, how many people are sick, and how many people die, and so we have to use the reported numbers we have and what is known about diseases to estimate and model these numbers.

In the real world with real diseases, there's a huge problem with detecting infections that don't cause serious illnesses. If we don't know everyone who is infected, it makes it hard to calculate the infection fatality rate. Typically, people don't get tested and treated for a disease unless they're sick, often quite grievously so. And therefore, in our minds, we tend to equate viruses with infections, and all infections with some form of disease. We don't worry about asymptomatic cases of infections with influenza: if someone isn't sick, we assume they haven't been infected at all. For many people, this is the first time in their lives that they're having to think about the possibility of silent infections and spread.

Asymptomatic people have limited compulsion to get tested for any disease. For SARS-CoV-2, knowledge of close interactions and contact of everyone who has come in contact with a known case may cause us to sit up and notice for the first time in our lives what is a fairly routine occurrence.

Now, let's think about the symptoms of COVID-19 themselves—they're broad and fairly non-specific. Chances are even if you haven't been tested yet with the SARS-CoV-2 you've wondered if you've been infected if you've even had a mild cough. That's because the list of symptoms for most respiratory infectious diseases are overlapping.

A person with mild sickness may not get tested because she doesn't know that the cough she has been suffering from is a symptom of COVID-19 and not a symptom of the flu or another respiratory disease. That doesn't mean the SARS-CoV-2 is the flu or common cold. Even if you think some countries have overreacted, the data will show you that this is not the flu. When all the data comes in on how many people are infected but didn't know, the infection fatality ratio is going to be less than 1 per cent, but probably in the range of twenty times worse than a seasonal flu strain.[1]

What happens early in an epidemic is that cases that are most severe and follow a narrowly defined definition of disease are reported. These are the people who are tested and they're also more likely to die. So, an early case fatality rate is more likely to be higher. This is something that was observed with the 2009 H1N1 influenza pandemic as well, when we overestimated the case fatality rate. As more cases become known, the case fatality rate falls.

It is difficult to calculate these numbers during a pandemic. Early on, an official of the WHO indicated that the case fatality rate was on the order of 4 per cent, which would make it more severe than the pandemic influenza of 1918. The symptoms used to narrow down people eligible for testing were serious at the time. The criteria for diagnosing the disease were very narrow.

In fact, the case fatality for Wuhan was higher than for the rest of China because of another reason. The fatality of a disease depends on how prepared people are to face a disease. If there is a shortage of critical care hospital beds, drugs and supplies, there will be a higher fatality. Over time, more is known about the disease and more treatment options for those who are seriously ill become available. This results in a drop in mortality.

One other point to remember is that confirmed deaths must be *attributed* to COVID-19 and confirmed cases must have a true positive test for SARS-CoV-2. Those with an active infection can be tested by RT-PCR. Those who were infected in the past will require an antibody test. A presumed COVID-19 fatality is not a confirmed COVID-19 fatality unless there is a diagnostic test to back up the diagnosis.

Molecular diagnostic tests such as RT-PCR were not available during some earlier pandemics, when public health specialists compared peak excess deaths. This can be done for COVID-19 as well where testing is inadequate, and clusters are suspected. In fact, in parts of Africa and South America, where testing reagents were in short supply, excess deaths were used to estimate the magnitude of local outbreaks.

The case fatality ranges from 1 per cent in some countries to around 15 per cent in others.[2] Some of these may be due to actual differences and some others due to limitations in calculating cases.

With all these comparisons in mind, the best estimates of the US CDC for the case fatality rate hover between 0.2 per cent and 1 per cent with a likelihood of around 0.4 per cent.[3] What that means is across a broad population there is a one in 250 chance that someone who is sick with COVID-19 will die from the disease. However, the case fatality rate steeply climbs with age. Someone under the age of fifty may have a 1 in 2000 chance of dying, which climbs to one in 500 for someone between the ages of fifty and sixty-four, and to one in seventy-five in those above sixty-five.

A broadly similar age-specific fatality rate has been observed for two Indian states, except for those above seventy-five: in these two Indian states, mortality plateaued under sixty-five.[4]

Early on, the WHO noted that there were very few cases of COVID-19 in children.[5] They seem to be spared. This is quite different from influenza strains in which children are often the drivers of infection, though they have mild disease. School closings are a targeted measure for controlling influenza, so they were adopted for SARS-CoV-2 as a precautionary step.

This is akin to what has been observed for other coronaviruses. Human coronaviruses that cause colds infect children multiple times a year causing niggling colds. During the SARS epidemic, of those who died, none was under the age of twenty-four.[6] On the other hand, over half the people diagnosed with SARS over the age of sixty-five died. A study in *Science* suggested that children might have some cross-reactive antibodies from previous cold-causing coronavirus infections that offer protection from SARS-CoV-2 infection.[7] However, further examination of this theory is warranted.

Hospitalization of children is relatively rare. Under 7 per cent of children admitted to hospitals require breathing support. A rare multi-inflammatory syndrome in children has been reported from Europe and North America and is found in one in 50,000 people under the age of twenty-one.[8]

Are children less susceptible to infection, or are they more likely to harbour silent infections? It is likely that it is a bit of both. A modelling study estimated that individuals under the age of twenty are half as likely to be infected as adults over that age.[9] Only around one in five of those between the ages of ten to nineteen who do get infected develop symptomatic COVID-19. All other things being equal, countries with younger populations can therefore be expected to have fewer mortalities than those with aging populations. However, children can spread infections to others in their households.

The impact of school closures on spread of SARS-CoV-2 has been difficult to gauge through 2020 because many children harbour silent infections and the infectiousness of children compared to adults remains mostly unknown.[10] However, a large-scale study of children in Andhra Pradesh and Tamil Nadu, India, found high prevalence of infection, suggesting school closures may have been warranted.

Observations made during the two major influenza pandemics of the twentieth century reinforce the thesis that schoolchildren are important in the spread of influenza. Even though the populations were universally susceptible to the new influenza viruses that emerged in 1918 and 1957, and even though both viruses had seeded the population in the preceding spring and summer, the first major wave did not occur until schools were in session. Peak activity of both pandemics occurred in late October after schools had been in session for six to eight weeks. School closures were also strongly associated with slowing the spread of influenza during the 2009 pandemic.

What about people with underlying conditions who have COVID-19? Older patients have declining immune responses, but also other health conditions or *comorbidities* such as heart disease, high blood pressure, cancer and diabetes. The risk of fatality among these populations is highest. Among the infected, those who are obese are twice as likely to be hospitalized and more than 50 per cent likely to die than those who are not.[11] Pregnant women are more likely to be hospitalized than women of similar age who are not.[12]

Sex also matters. Females are less likely to die than males. Part of it stems from behavioural aspects—women are more likely to consider the pandemic serious and comply with preventative measures.[13] But it isn't simply that men make riskier choices or suffer from other underlying conditions. It is likely that there are actual differences in immune responses.[14]

At the time of writing, more research is needed on risk factors such as race, poverty, ethnicity and health structure. Are there genetic factors and predispositions or are difference in fatality rates because of a combination of underlying health practices, lack of services, greater exposure and malnutrition?

A study found that a genetic region found in some (but not all people) increased the susceptibility to serious COVID-19 in those who were infected. The study also found that this gene region, inherited from Neanderthals, can be found in around 50 per cent of the people of South Asia, including Pakistan, India and Bangladesh. But how this Neanderthal component can be reconciled with other factors such as age, existing conditions and general immunity is unknown.[15]

In December, a study published in *Nature* found that there were at least five genes tied to immunity and inflammation that put people at a greater risk of more serious outcomes of COVID-19.[16] But targeting those genes to effectively prevent those outcomes seems at least years away.

# 16

# Infectiousness

Although most people use 'infectious' and 'contagious' synonymously in everyday parlance, there's a difference in what they actually mean. Infectious diseases are those that can be transmitted directly by humans and animals, or indirectly by means of contaminated objects or vectors of disease (insects or larger animals). A contagious disease is one that is spread directly between humans and there's no need for an indirect route. Malaria is an infectious disease, but it's not contagious since it doesn't spread directly from one person to another; there's a requirement for mosquito vectors in between. All contagious diseases are infectious, but the opposite isn't true. SARS-CoV-2 is both infectious and contagious. Most transmission is from one human to another.

How infectious is the SARS-CoV-2? Unless you have been in a cave since the middle of January 2020, you already know that the answer to that is 'very'. But how much is important since this is a central part of the story.

Several factors determine the course of a pandemic, but one of the most important is the basic reproduction number (R0, pronounced as R-naught). This number gives a sense of the average number of people who are infected by one person in a population that is susceptible to infection. Because this is such a central concept to everything we know about COVID-19, it's important to break this down.

First, a word about the name. Sometimes R0 is called the basic reproduction rate, but strictly speaking it is not a rate that has a unit. It doesn't tell us how fast an infection is spreading or how severe the symptoms are. Even in a scene in the blockbuster Hollywood movie *Contagion*, an epidemiologist played by Kate Winslet goes up to the whiteboard and scribbles a few diseases referring to the numbers next to them as basic reproductive rates (it's a riveting movie, nonetheless).

The idea of the reproduction number originated outside the field of epidemiology. Demographer Alfred Lotka conceived of the R0 in the 1920s, as a means of measuring the number of offspring in a given population. Later, in the 1950s, epidemiologist George MacDonald advocated using it as a measure of the spread of malaria.

Researchers also use the R0 as a means of thinking of the number of people one person will infect in the absence of measures to stop spread. For a population, this can be used to figure out the maximum pandemic potential of a virus in a setting. It is a baseline from which we can estimate the relative effectiveness of separate interventions such as school closures, work from home and distancing.

An R0 for an infectious disease at a place is generally reported as a single numeric value or range. R0 is not an internal property of the infectious agent but is characteristic of the agent acting within a specific host within a given setting. In other words, the value depends on many factors.

Let's lay the foundation for a new disease like COVID-19. We are considering a situation in which one person who is infected is in a population in which theoretically there is no one with immunity, or in other words, everyone is susceptible. The formal definition of the R0 of a disease is the number of cases, on average, an infected person will cause during their infectious period.

The R0 for SARS-CoV-2 is predicted to be between 2 and 3 in most settings. That means one person on average infects two to three more (though 'super-spreading' situations where one person infects more than the average complicates matters).

How does this compare with the R0 for other diseases? For almost all strains of the seasonal flu, it is between 1 and 2. For pandemic influenza, it is often higher; for example, for the H1N1 1918 influenza pandemic it has been calculated as being between 2.2 and 2.9 which is similar to the R0 for SARS-CoV-2 under most situations.

For the SARS epidemic of 2002 and 2003, scientists estimated the original R0 was around 2.75. But even after the R0 dropped below 1 (thanks to the tremendous effort that went into isolation and quarantine), the virus raged on. This is because as long as susceptible individuals are present in large numbers, spread may continue. Even when a virus has a low R0 there are situations such as crowding that may cause spread.

Let's think of a new virus that causes an infectious disease in terms of those who are susceptible to the disease, those who are infected and those who have recovered. At first, for a disease for which there is no immunity, everyone will be in the susceptible compartment. Over time, more people will get infected, and then they will recover (or perish). As the virus spreads like fire, over time more people get infected and become immune, and these people may become dead ends for getting reinfected and further spreading the disease. What also prevents the disease from dying out is the addition of new susceptible people to the population, mainly from new births.

As an epidemic progresses, the basic reproduction number gives way to the effective reproduction number which declines until it falls below 1 in value. The epidemic then decays, either due to the exhaustion of people susceptible to infection, or because of the success of control measures.

Although R0 is an important number, it is usually an estimate based on mathematical calculations. The three main considerations are how long someone is infectious for after they've become infected, the contact rate and the chance of infection of each contact during this time. All other things being equal, a virus that causes people to be infectious for a week is going to cause more secondary infections than one that is infectious for a day.

Gregarious people in a densely populated city may encounter a lot of people. And the duration for which someone who has a silent infection and is mobile and unwittingly infecting others may be different from someone who has symptomatic COVID-19 and is isolated in a hospital. These are just some of the factors that make an accurate calculation difficult in the middle of a pandemic.

What may be clear is that the reproduction number isn't completely a property of the virus. It also depends on the environment and it depends on people. And that's why measures are also important. The goal of public health measures is to keep the effective reproduction number as far below 1 as possible, because once measures are relaxed, it will rise again. In 2020, world leaders such as Angela Merkel, the chancellor of Germany, frequently quoted the calculated reproduction number under the influence of various measures.[1]

Scientists calculated that the start of the outbreak in Wuhan, when the agent wasn't known and there were no measures in place, one person was infecting (on average) more than three other people. Strict suppression including the lockdown instituted in Wuhan on 23 January 2020 brought the effective reproduction number down to 0.67 by 8 March.[2]

With a higher reproduction number, there may be recommendations for greater measures such as social distancing or lockdowns to reduce the number of contacts. A higher reproduction number also means that declines due to seasonal effects might not end an epidemic, only slow it down somewhat.

R0 can also be used to get an idea of how many people might be infected in a susceptible population if no effective measures are taken. This fraction can be calculated by a simple formula

(1–1/ R0). If R0 values for COVID-19 are around 2.5, that means that 60 per cent of the population may need to become infected to confer herd immunity. If the R0 is 2.2, this threshold is only 55 per cent. But at an R0, of 5.7, this threshold rises to 82 per cent. The higher the R0, the more the number of people who need to be infected to get to herd immunity.

I should mention that this formula does not provide a completely accurate calculation of herd immunity, because not everyone is susceptible at the start of a pandemic. There is some debate as to how often children get infected compared to adults. One study found that children may be infected at 50 per cent of the rate as adults. Another found that those under ten may also pass the virus less efficiently. It's not clear how susceptible other groups in a large population are either. It's conceivable that some people might have some antibodies from infections from other viruses that confer some immunity. Also, there's the open question of trained immunity induced by BCG vaccination. Are populations that have received BCG vaccines in childhood less susceptible to SARS-CoV-2 infection? Some scientists certainly think so, though the ultimate proof will come from controlled experiments with the vaccine.

## Superspreaders

The importance of the R0 in understanding pandemics and in formulating public health policy is paramount. It is conceptually easy to grasp and to visualize. With an R0 of 3, I can draw a simple tree with branches representing each person and visualize three additional branches sprouting from each point. I can keep doing this and get a sense of the extent of exponential spread. If a lockdown is instituted early, and social distancing occurs, I'll know that many of those earlier branches will not give rise to more branches.

A really big assumption is that there are no major variations in how the individual people in the population spread the disease.

I'm assuming that every person in the scenario of an R0 of 3 is going to infect three more people. But what if this were not true? What if people didn't have an equal chance of transmitting disease?

For certain diseases in specific outbreak locations, there can be people who are so-called *super-spreaders*, who transmit infections onto many more people than the average.[3] On the flipside, in this scenario there are a lot of people who are not spreading infections at all. There's something called the 20/80 rule in which 20 per cent of the people who are most infectious are responsible for 80 per cent of the spread of the disease.[4] Superspreading has been known to occur for sexually transmitted diseases such as HIV/AIDS. One of the first times superspreading was truly appreciated for a coronavirus was with SARS. For SARS, even after the reproduction number was lowered below 1, the virus kept spreading because of a few people spreading to many.

One of the most significant conclusions of a large analysis of SARS-CoV-2 transmission in two Indian states was that not all infected people were spreading the virus: in fact, most people weren't. As much as 71 per cent of reported cases had not spread the virus to anyone else.[5] And less than 10 per cent of people transmitted nearly two-thirds of identified infections.[6]

Not all virus outbreaks have superspreaders and superspreading events. The spread of Ebola during the 2000 outbreak in Uganda was remarkably consistent in terms of how many secondary infections were caused by each infected person. Superspreaders are also uncommon with influenza.

When there are few people infected at a place in the initial stages of an infection, certain events can determine the trajectory of the epidemic. The effect of superspreading events in Korea, Italy and in India is well documented.[7]

Major outbreaks of SARS-CoV-2 occurred in correctional facilities among incarcerated populations.[8] It is incorrect to think of jails as closed systems. Correctional officers travel home and elsewhere and return. When restricting freedom to closely confined spaces takes precedence, social distancing is not a priority. Outbreaks are rapid as exposure is caught late. Cleaning agents, masks and other protective measures are often not available in sufficient quantities.

Major clusters of infections worldwide were also observed at meatpacking plants where low temperatures allow the virus to survive, nursing homes where there are susceptible elderly populations, and at gatherings where crowds formed such as the Biogen Conference in the US, Shincheonji Church of Jesus outside Seoul, and at weddings and funerals. Cruise ships and navy vessels, including the aircraft carrier of the *USS Theodore Roosevelt*, were the source of outbreaks. Bars and restaurants in Tokyo and in other cities also witnessed outbreaks.

What can we do to prevent spread based on this knowledge? We don't know yet who is going to be a superspreader and who is not. Avoiding crowds and clusters in indoor settings such as restaurants and gyms is the best way to avoid superspreading events.

## Seasonality

During the first few months of the pandemic many of us received questionable claims that COVID-19 would vanish in the summer months. Some of these theories were based on influenza and the common cold. There's a problem with trying to extrapolate from established viruses that cause seasonal diseases to new viruses that cause pandemics. There's some immunity to endemic diseases and little to none to new ones.

People have known about seasonal variations in the spread of respiratory infectious diseases for thousands of years, much before the causes of these diseases were known. Colloquially, in English and in Indian languages, we refer to diseases caused by certain viruses that cause outbreaks in winters as 'catching a cold'. Seasonal fluctuations in spread have been observed for a lot of common respiratory infectious diseases and the phenomenon is called *seasonality*. We typically observe the flu season starting in October and November to April in the northern hemisphere. Likewise, human coronaviruses cause colds from December to April.

Despite being one of the most well-known phenomena, especially with respect to influenza which has a huge global disease burden, it is only recently that we've made progress in deciphering what the actual reasons might be for so-called seasonality. Humidity may play a role. The relative humidity declines in the winter months. Temperature is also thought to impact seasonality.

In affluent countries, there is indoor heating in winter and air-conditioning in summer. People in affluent countries spend around 90 per cent of their time indoors, and this has significant implications for disease spread.[9] People are breathing the same air and getting less fresh air than their ancestors.

What should give us pause is that even influenza viruses that cause major pandemics behave differently from seasonal influenza strains. Of the ten or so pandemics in the last 250 years caused by influenza viruses, all had second waves around six months from the first regardless of the season they started in. Many of the influenza pandemics originate in tropical climates and regions with year-round elevated temperature.

SARS-CoV-2 has a lower stability at higher temperatures and higher humidity, a characteristic the virus shares with other human coronaviruses, SARS coronavirus and influenza viruses. But this was not adequate to make the virus go away completely in the summer. Conversely, SARS-CoV-2 infections did rebound in Europe and North America in the autumn and winter of 2020.[10] What the relative effects of atmosphere temperature and humidity are compared to more people staying indoors was unknown at the time of writing.

Incidentally, since influenza spreads in much the same way as SARS-CoV-2 does, one of the effects of much of the world locking down in March is that the flu season in the northern hemisphere was cut short by roughly six weeks. In the fall and winter of 2020, fewer cases of flu were also reported in the northern hemisphere.

# 17

# Measures

Although often used synonymously, isolation and quarantine are not the same thing. Those who have been positively identified as infected are *isolated* so that they don't spread the virus. They may be isolated in wards in hospitals or at home (sometimes with a device that checks oxygen levels, a pulse oximeter).

A *quarantine* involves restricting movements of someone who may have come in contact with an infected person or object for a certain amount of time (usually similar to longest incubation period normally observed) to see if they get sick. If they get sick or are infected, they go into isolation. Quarantine laws also apply to people who enter a country or an area from one where there is an active outbreak or cluster of infections. The quarantine period for SARS-CoV-2 was set at fourteen days because most people who got sick developed symptoms before that time. Most people were not infectious after eight days either, so fourteen days was a reasonable amount of time to control spread in most cases.

The original idea of quarantine (which derives from 'quaranta', the word for forty) comes from the fourteenth-century practice of holding ships for thirty, and later forty, days outside Dubrovnik, Venice and Milan to protect them from plague epidemics. Quarantine laws applied not only to people but also to goods. Quarantine measures have remained a cornerstone of disease-control measures because they are effective. Quarantines have been imposed in India for over a century and have not always been received kindly. The 1897 Epidemic Diseases Act instituted during a plague epidemic prompted violence because it allowed women to be isolated in quarantine camps. Plague commissioner W.C. Rand was assassinated in June of that year in Pune. Rioting broke out across much of India the following year protesting plague quarantines.

Quarantines have been used during this pandemic as well. One of the most famous examples in 2020 was the quarantine of all passengers on the *Diamond Princess* cruise ship outside the Japanese port city of Yokohama. This quarantine was criticized for not stopping the spread of the disease. Over 700 people out of 3711 were infected. In February 2020, this accounted for a substantial number of known infections outside of China.

## Containment

At the start of an outbreak the goal is to be able to contain spread by identifying every single infected person and who they've come in contact with. Containment depends on the ability to identify the infected early, isolate them and trace those they have contacted. The goal of containment is to keep the outbreak under check so that it doesn't become unmanageable. Diagnostic testing paired with isolation early in an infection is effective, especially when someone may be spreading germs without knowing it. Even a delay of a day when someone is infectious may cause them to infect many others. Once a positive case is confirmed, the person is isolated. Everyone who has come into contact is 'traced' using both electronic and in-person measures: those who have come in contact are quarantined.

There are several factors (including luck) that determine the spread of a disease. Even one large outbreak can cause a shift in measures taken. However, if a community employs containment strategy early and aggressively, and the population is compliant in following control measures, this approach may be more successful and impose less limitations on movement compared to other measures.

Containment is difficult for a virus that causes 'silent infections' among people who can transmit the virus to others who might get sick. Contact tracing is an arduous process. Mobile apps can help, but often some in-person intervention is required. Because the infectiousness of SARS-CoV-2 is greatest early in infection at a time when many people harbour silent infections, they may be moving around infecting other people. Minimizing delays in testing have the greatest effect on preventing onward transmission. When paired with effective tracing that integrated app-based technology provides, a substantial proportion of subsequent transmissions may be prevented. But it's not easy. It is estimated that seven out of ten contacts must be traced early for containment to be successful.

At the end of September, the largest contact tracing study to date had been published with data from Andhra Pradesh and Tamil Nadu. Contact tracers in these two states had reached out to over 3 million contacts of 435,539 cases, but full testing data was available on around 575,000 contacts exposed to nearly 85,000 confirmed positive cases of SARS-CoV-2.[1]

## Mitigation

There is a tipping point when diagnostic testing, isolating confirmed positive cases and contact tracing of those who might be infected are no longer manageable with available resources or effective in controlling spread. Containment works until cases start popping up everywhere. When containment is no longer effective, and multiple clusters of infection and community spread have been observed, the community may need to employ mitigation. At this point broader school and business closures may be necessary.

Social-distancing measures such as cancelling conferences, sporting events and other large gatherings are implemented. The aim of mitigation is to reduce spread while protecting the most vulnerable people. Infections will continue to rage on until a sizable portion of the population has been protected by a vaccine or by herd immunity.

No country has a healthcare system designed to treat all patients in an unmitigated out-of-control pandemic. Mitigation ensures that surge capacity is never met, that all who are sick can get treated and that instruments such as mechanical ventilators that help sick people breathe are available. We know that when a healthcare system is overrun with patients, the fatality rate increases. This was observed in Wuhan, China, and in Lombardy, Italy, in the first few months of the outbreak. If a healthcare system is saturated, deaths can also occur from other causes, a situation that was observed during the Ebola outbreak of 2014-15 in West Africa.

The goal of mitigation is ultimately to flatten the epidemic curve. Doing so also allows scientific discoveries to be made, vaccines and drugs to be tested and developed, modes of transmission to be discovered, the effectiveness of measures to be tested and drugs to be manufactured at scale.

As we learned for the COVID-19 pandemic, identifying the optimal time for initiating measures can be difficult.[2] However, countries which were affected later learn from the experiences of countries which were impacted earlier. For planning purposes for influenza, it was recommended that interventions be kept for a maximum of three months, depending on the severity of the pandemic virus.

The effectiveness of mitigation strategies has been studied in detail for cities in the United States that had been impacted by the H1N1 influenza pandemic in 1918 and 1919.[3] Broadly, cities that employed many measures and kept them in place without succumbing to fatigue saved the most lives. Both the time and the duration of the deployment of measures seem to be crucial.

We need to make educated predictions, known as *models*. Models are a way to predict what may happen based on assumptions that are known to be valid at the time. As assumptions change, so do models. A model can't account for everything that may impact the future outcome: there would simply be too many variables. Scientists come up with different models all the time and there can be rigorous, heated disagreement on their validity. But the point to remember is that while a model is a simple framework, what it describes, in this case the spread of disease, is very real. And in the case of a pandemic, different models have shaped all our lives.

Some epidemiological models of a pandemic give worst-case scenarios of how many may get infected and may die. In a perfect world, scientists would have ample time to test out all assumptions while building their models to be able to make more accurate predictions. But in the real world, there is a need to act with alacrity during a pandemic and to formulate measures that control the spread of infections. Ironically, if the measures that are proposed end up being too successful, the worst-case scenario never comes to pass and not as many people are infected or die as predicted: by virtue of reacting, the doomsday scenario never happens. What happens in this case is that many people doubt whether the measures were necessary in the first place!

Based on a model created by using human coronaviruses, a group of researchers predicted that social-distancing measures may be necessary into 2022 to prevent hospital capacity from being exceeded.[4] If there's post-infection immunity, the study predicted that the virus might be gone for five years or more. If there's no post-infection immunity, the virus will become endemic in humans.

It should be noted that measures don't have to be perfect to be successful and 100 per cent compliance is never achievable.

However, by breaking chains of transmission and preventing clusters, spread is kept to manageable proportions.

The question of how long the COVID-19 pandemic will last is a tricky one. In the absence of broad vaccination of populations or a game-changing drug that is effective in 90 per cent or more of the people who need it most, a pandemic that ends rapidly due to mass infection and death may be the worst possible outcome. Mitigation slows down spread. As such, paradoxically it actually prolongs a pandemic, allowing vaccination to offer more benign protection than that resulting from infection. An unmitigated pandemic ends quicker than a mitigated one. Herd immunity is acquired more rapidly. But in the process, there are many more deaths. I know this is counterintuitive when we want a pandemic to end rapidly. But *how* a pandemic ends is important.

## Suppression

Researchers modified a computer model developed for flu pandemic simulations for SARS-CoV-2.[5] They found that even with the best mitigation scenario consisting of case isolation, home quarantine and social distancing for the elderly, healthcare systems would be overwhelmed and millions of people would die. Subsequently, some of the assumptions of this influential model were refined, but the broad conclusions remained unchanged.

There is one more option, and that is one of last resort, suppression. Suppression brings a hammer down to stop the spread of the virus. The measures are stronger than mitigation because they include social distancing of the *entire* population. An example of suppression is the lockdown that Wuhan instituted on 23 January 2020.

Of course, in a large and heterogeneous country, suppression is harder to maintain and enforce. One part of the country may obtain compliance from the population. However, another may hastily open and see a resurgence in infections. Like mitigation, suppression slows the spread of the disease but does not eradicate it. It addresses an acute problem. Like mitigation, suppression also pushes the curve into the future. And while it is an extremely aggressive measure, when it is successful, it also makes up for lost time by resetting the clock. Once spread has been suppressed, the goal is to slowly allow normal activities to resume with careful surveillance. If suppression is a hammer, what follows is a dance. Whenever cases flare up, containment zones are created, and isolating and contact tracing are performed until all cases can be identified. Many experts predict that many rounds of suppression and lifting of measures will be required until a vaccine can be administered broadly.

A research team modelled the impact of a five-month suppression scenario and calculated the reduction of deaths.[6] The team found that the best strategy to control SARS-CoV-2 would involve isolation of those who are infected, quarantine of members of households of those who are infected, social distancing of the entire population and shutting down all schools and universities. They predicted that though there would be a second wave of cases, suppression would be, by far, the best strategy. This model was very influential in forcing the UK to employ suppression tactics, after flirting with the idea of a quicker herd immunity through less restrictive measures. This model also influenced the US to implement stay-at-home orders in March. Lastly, the authors anticipated that countries would struggle to maintain a suppression model for the duration of time needed to control infections. The authors suggested that suppression may need to continue for a year-and-a-half. Realizing that a lockdown of this duration is impractical, the authors suggested that at least the elderly should be sequestered from the rest of the population.

When population-level social distancing should be applied is a matter for debate. But a trigger is when there are significant clusters of infection and community transmission. In addition, the rise in cases can be examined and plotted: if it is exponential with cases doubling every few days, managing infections using non-suppression tactics is difficult.

A lockdown is a large-scale mandated closure involving orders to stay at home and to limit movement. It is the key differentiating factor between suppression and mitigation. In some jurisdictions, lockdowns are called shutdowns and in others, shelter-in-place orders. Many types of measures of differing restrictions and compliances fall under a vague 'lockdown'—from a laissez-faire lockdown based on a code of honour with lax enforcement, to a restrictive closure with strict fines and imprisonment. For example, the US never formally had a lockdown—there was a stay-at-home order that was very loosely enforced by different states. India, on the other hand, had a more stringent lockdown that was praised by the WHO.[7]

European nations instituted a second series of measures for a few weeks in October 2020.[8] While in many cases, these measures were not as severe as the first lockdowns in March, they did involve closing restaurants and bars, restricting public gatherings and mandating the wearing of facemasks. The UK implemented heightened measures prior to Christmas in response to concerns over the possible rapid spread of a new variant of SARS-CoV-2.[9]

Most lockdowns involve cessation of business activities outside of the home. Those who work in essential services such as healthcare, essential transportation and infrastructure, and governance are exempted, though the definition of essential services also varies significantly from country to country. When a lockdown was first instituted in Belgium, bookstores and potato-fries stands remained open. In France, wine shops and tobacconists were exempted. In the Netherlands, marijuana was still legally available. In some countries, there were exceptions for outdoor activities so long as social distance was maintained.

If deciding when to institute a lockdown is problematic, figuring out when to loosen one is contentious.[10] Expert guidelines suggest loosening a lockdown after observing two weeks of declining cases; confirming that there are adequate hospital and diagnostic testing capacity; and determining that there is adequate contact tracing capacity. Suppression can result in a situation in which the average number of infections resulting from one infected person falls below 1. But according to health experts, suppression should be maintained as much as feasible, because cases will rise once again once extreme measures are removed.

Ultimately, there are social, economic and political factors that determine when suppression strategies are loosened. Fatigue sets in, especially after tens of millions of jobs are lost. The ability to sustain and support measures (on an individual level) often comes from a position of privilege that not everyone possesses.

# 18

# Effectiveness

What measures worked for the first surge of the pandemic?

Imagine that the world was in suspended animation for a few months. Everyone would freeze in place, metabolize and wake up later with no recollection of what had happened. Let us also ignore what would happen to the vast infrastructure of the world created by humans and imagine everything remained intact. In that time, with every human frozen in place, the virus would have no way to transmit from one human to another and would come close to eradication. There is always the possibility that someone may remain infectious for an abnormally long time, and that it might linger on some cold surfaces. There's also the possibility that the virus might spread in animals like cats and monkeys and reinfect people later. But the broader purpose of indulging in this exercise is to understand how the virus is usually spread. SARS-CoV-2 is spread by people.

The closest option to 'freezing' the planet is the lockdown that was undertaken in Wuhan, where the city and province were closed off from the rest of the country and everyone except for the essential workers and the sick stayed indoors for two months. A strict lockdown is nearly 100 per cent effective in stopping spread provided it is implemented fully and early. Of course, a full lockdown with millions of people is extremely difficult to achieve everywhere. Lockdowns are different in different places. For example, the lockdown in the United States in March is thought to have been half as strict as the first lockdowns in western Europe at the same time. Realistically, even a lockdown that achieves 75 per cent compliance is successful.

In a pandemic what we want to also know is what can keep transmission under control to return to normal life with minimum disruption. Unfortunately, there are no easy decisions. A four- or five-month complete lockdown with as many measures as possible might be best, but that comes at a price: economic destruction. Lockdowns for a protracted period of time are economically, socially and psychologically corrosive. They are a weapon of last resort because the costs are immense.

When multiple measures are layered together it is difficult to know their relative benefits. If testing, tracing and isolating regimens are relaxed after measures are lifted, there may be renewed outbreaks, so the benefits of the lockdown are soon forgotten. A mitigated or suppressed pandemic may last longer but will have fewer cases overall and fewer deaths. The slower acceleration should not be seen as failure since it also keeps healthcare facilities from being overrun. Treatment options are developed. Vaccines go into trials and then into production. The experience of 1918 is that most communities must institute some form of social-distancing measures but not all measures will be equally effective.

The second thing we need to look at are the measures themselves and how they rank. Oxford ran a COVID-19 government response tracker for thirteen interventions in more than 100 countries and compiled them into a stringency index that went from low to high. At the high end of the stringency index were countries like India and South Africa which were both initially praised for aggressive lockdowns.

A lot of how transmission occurs is dependent on the size of the country, population density, behaviour (such as willingness to wear facemasks), willingness to adhere to authority and national policy. The risk for a large country in which states and local governments exert control (such as India, Brazil and the United States) is different from a small country with strict national governance.

Additionally, the trajectory of spread can change very quickly. Some countries which had excellent responses initially experienced outbreaks by July. Singapore's outbreaks occurred in migrant dormitories. Outbreaks in Israel occurred in schools. Nightclubs and bars were the source of outbreaks in Japan and South Korea.

Still, some countries were extraordinarily successful in keeping the number of fatalities low through the first seven months of 2020. During this time Uganda, Vietnam, Laos, Mongolia and Cambodia had not reported a single death due to COVID-19. Rwanda, hailed as a model for many countries, had only four deaths through 11 July. It showed that it was possible to use pooled testing, clear leadership and boots-on-the-ground tracing to stay in containment.[1] Rwanda serves as an excellent example of how a low-income country, with limited resources, can stop the spread of infections. Rwanda solved the problem of expensive test reagents by pooling nasal swabs in one vial and testing multiple samples cost-effectively. If a sample tested positive, all the samples were individually tested. This process works when the prevalence is low and there are no clusters of outbreaks.

In Rwanda, any positive case was immediately isolated at a dedicated COVID-19 clinic. Health workers called or visited every potential contact of anyone who tested positive. Any contacts identified were also quarantined. Testing and treatment for COVID-19 were free. Rwanda mobilized community healthcare workers, police and college students to work as contact tracers. It set up national and regional command posts to track cases. It even used human-size robots in COVID-19 clinics to take patients' temperatures and deliver supplies.

Hong Kong had not instituted a lockdown in the first six months of the outbreak. In 2003, Hong Kong had suffered greatly from SARS and they learned from that experience. Authorities did not feel the need to institute a comprehensive lockdown because they took measures early. In January 2020, Hong Kong instituted restrictions at the border, the use of masks and other protective gear, social distancing, cleaning and aggressive isolation of cases along with identification of contacts and quarantine. Hong Kong did not try to identify which measure worked best but instead, assumed all contributed to their early success. In the ten weeks since the first patient with COVID-19 was identified, these measures resulted in very low transmission. With good compliance from the public, transparent communication, an epidemiological plan, and aggressive testing, tracing and isolating, Hong Kong was able to prevent the disease from blowing out of proportion through June. But it was not out of the woods completely and suffered what was called a 'third wave' of infections in July, which was contained by September.

The government of South Korea relied on large-scale disinfection, massive testing, tracing of those who had been contacted by infected people and quarantine. In what seems like shocking prescient timing, South Korea had drilled for a potential coronavirus epidemic in December 2019.[2] Two dozen infectious disease specialists planned for a scenario in which many cases of pneumonia would strike the country. Korea was hit early because of outbreaks associated with a person who spread the virus at Shincheonji Church in Daegu in February 2020. By late February, South Korea had drive-through testing centres and was testing 10,000 people daily. The public readily cooperated with measures and facemasks were also distributed. Despite the speed of the outbreak, South Korea had not instituted a full-scale lockdown in 2020, though some businesses were closed. After some social-distancing restrictions were relaxed in May, there were outbreaks in nightclubs in Seoul, prompting new restrictions to be put in place.

Japan built its strategy of preventing infections around modification of behaviour, asking its citizens to avoid the 'three Cs' of closed spaces, crowded places and close-contact settings.[3] Researchers in Japan predicted that the risk of infections indoors might be nineteen times higher than outdoors. Tokyo is more than two times as densely populated as New York City. And yet through mid-July, Tokyo had experienced only a fraction of cases of New York City. By focusing on clusters of infections, Japan was able to prevent superspreading events. Japan has a high percentage of people over sixty-five, but it was able to protect them from infections. From a public health perspective, Japan also relied on early detection and response, but in contrast to South Korea, did not depend on mass testing. But even this strategy had limitations. Japan realized that its cluster-control strategy was insufficient when there was another surge in November.

Report after report highlighted the need to act early and decisively. Germany and Austria took an early aggressive approach, compared to Italy, Spain and France which took a much laxer attitude to control and social distancing until the epidemic had caused many more deaths. Germany had a lower per capita rate of infections than those countries through most of 2020. It sequentially cancelled large events, closed schools and then instituted social distancing. A study showed that all the measures were necessary to reduce spread, though the closure of schools and business was predicted to have the greatest impact.[4] Effects of measures were detected about two weeks after application. The impact on deaths could be detected a week or two after that.

In Europe, algorithms group Sweden, the United Kingdom and the Netherlands together as countries that acted relatively slowly through early 2020. In the initial stages of the pandemic, all three implemented 'herd immunity' strategies, which involved fewer measures, or ones that rely on voluntary compliance.

Later, the United Kingdom and the Netherlands switched to more aggressive responses, including country-wide lockdown. These two countries also instituted a second less-restrictive lockdown later in the year. On the other hand, with the virus rampant through the country and deaths piling up, Sweden was forced to reassess its approach in November.

A draconian lockdown results in massive disruption and is difficult to manage. Compliance in large countries with varied demographics and healthcare system is problematic. Early findings from a research team suggest that poorer nations tended to bring in stricter measures than did richer countries, compared to the severity of their outbreaks. But conversely, many countries that did not control spread simply did not test fast enough (within twenty-four hours of suspicion) or broadly enough. The WHO recommends that countries should be able to control spread and have suitable systems to test, trace, and isolate so that healthcare systems aren't overwhelmed. By mid-May, more than 150 countries had not met the criterion of being able to reduce spread to clusters.

A large analysis reported on countries or regions that implemented restrictions on mass gatherings, lockdowns, closures of schools, closures of workplaces and closures of public transport in the first half of 2020.[5] All 149 countries applied three out of five measures between 1 January and 30 May 2020. All five measures were in place in 118 countries, including in India. Implementation of any physical-distancing measure was tied to 13 per cent reduction in incidence. An earlier application of a lockdown resulted in a greater reduction in new COVID-19 cases. Closure of public transport had the least effect. This is intuitive. If a region is under lockdown and schools and colleges are closed, people are less likely to use public transport in large numbers.

The study also found that the effect of physical-distancing measures was greatest in regions that were better prepared from a healthcare perspective, had an older population and greater overall income as measured by GDP. Reasons for this are unknown, but we can speculate. A low-income country without a social safety net and many people in the informal sector may have a more challenging time in obtaining and maintaining compliance. This is in line with the early results on the lockdowns and other associated measures on the restrictions of movement in Wuhan.

The lessons from the COVID-19 pandemic are that measures when layered, applied early and until clusters of infection can be controlled result in a flattened epidemic curve. This is consistent with what researchers had observed earlier. In 1918–19, early implementation and layering of measures such as quarantine and isolation, restrictions on public gatherings and school closures were associated with fewer deaths. And although the economy took a hit in regions that implemented aggressive measures early, they also grew faster after the pandemic ended.

## India locks down

The first positive case in India was reported on 30 January 2020. India repatriated many of its citizens from China and other countries and closed its borders. The country announced a lockdown of 1.3 billion people on 24 March, the largest experiment of its kind on a national scale. Initially, the lockdown was for twenty-one days (three weeks), but it was extended to 17 May. The country was praised by the WHO for its 'tough and timely' national lockdown and shutting of borders.[6] While the number of reported cases of SARS-CoV-2 infections in India was relatively small prior to the lockdown, the trajectory of exponential growth portended a major loss of life.

On 26 March, a day after the lockdown was initiated, an MRC Centre for Global Infectious Disease Analysis report described a mathematical model for the effects of various suppression strategies, including lockdowns.[7] The Centre predicted that over 250 days, in an unmitigated scenario in which countries in South Asia went on with business as usual, there would be 1.7 billion infections and 7.6 million deaths. This would be a tragedy unimaginable in scale since the 1918 pandemic. Criticisms of the model have been pointed out, and in fact the heterogeneity of various populations, actual susceptibility and variations in mortality among various age groups make this a worst-case scenario. Experts also noted that the lockdown would push the pandemic into the future and that a lockdown should only be used to build up testing and tracing capacity.

The lockdown, which was thought of as one of the most stringent in the world, did initially slow the spread of the epidemic. In India, the curve wasn't flattened, but the slope of the epidemic curve was altered. It has been calculated that the basic reproduction number for India was 2.08: due to measures taken during the lockdown, the effective reproduction number fell to 1.16 on 22 April.[8] From 20 April, states began to ease some of the restrictions that had been imposed and took the approach of demarcating hotspots of infections in containment zones. India also expanded the ability to test, trace and isolate.

In the first six months of 2020, India was relatively successful in controlling spread and minimizing death, given the size of the nation. In its favour is its relatively young population: around two-thirds of India's population is under the age of thirty-five and mortality is low in the young.

The lockdown was not without significant and sustained criticism, however. Some experts criticized the way the lockdown was initiated and its implementation as an administrative matter with little prior public intimation. And once the lockdown was loosened, cases began to spike. In much of September, India reported more daily new cases than any other country in the world.[9] Trailing the US, with over 10 million infected, India had the second highest number of reported cases of SARS-CoV-2 infection in 2020.[10]

India has millions of internal migrants. After the lockdown was instituted, hundreds of thousands of migrant workers embarked on an exodus from urban centres to their homes in villages and smaller towns, the largest internal movement of people since Partition in 1947.[11] They walked for hundred and even thousands of kilometres. Many succumbed to exhaustion, heat and starvation. By early May, it was claimed that more than 300 had died.[12]

During the lockdown, a vast gulf in social standing, economic inequalities and access to healthcare became apparent; while private hospitals charged exorbitant sums for a bed per night, migrants died of starvation and exhaustion as they tried to get home. The deaths of migrants remain the most vivid recollection of the lockdown in the minds of many. Amidst a barrage of news during the pandemic, a tragedy occurred on 8 May, when a freight train killed sixteen migrants who were resting on railway tracks near Aurangabad in Maharashtra.

Kerala was pointed out as a model to emulate early in 2020. The success of the state in stopping Nipah, using testing, contact tracing, information sharing and isolation came in handy in the first few months of the pandemic. Kerala fared better than many other states, in part because it has consistently spent money to build a world-class healthcare infrastructure, from training doctors and nurses to effective communication and community involvement.

Andhra Pradesh and Tamil Nadu were also pointed out as two states with relatively effective healthcare infrastructure compared to most of India. A large-scale study found that the number of secondary infections from one person declined by the third week of the lockdown, though calculating absolute numbers was difficult because of the increased testing during that timeframe.[13]

There is no doubt that the lockdown adversely affected India's economy. What has taken many observers by surprise is the extent of India's decline in GDP (by 23.9 per cent) in the June quarter of 2020.[14] India unveiled a fiscal stimulus plan in October, but many economists called for more robust fiscal support to stimulate consumption and alleviate poverty.[15]

An argument in favour of the lockdown is that it was necessary to save lives. A counterargument is that there are other countries with similar demographics that did a reasonable job in keeping infections (normalized by population) low without a similar decline in GDP.

The critical missing piece of information currently is how many lives were saved as a result of the lockdown. In other words, how many more people would have died in a no-lockdown situation? There is no direct way to compare the number of infections and deaths that would have occurred in a no-lockdown scenario with the current scenario for India, but such a scenario can be modelled. Many studies have been published in reputed journals such as *Science* and *Nature* for France, Germany, Europe and China (Wuhan and the rest of China) with similar data,[16] but through 2020, to the best of my knowledge, no such information was available for India.[17] For example, a study in *Nature* claims 3.1 million deaths were averted in eleven European countries due to measures taken.[18]

Another aspect of India's lockdown that warrants further investigation is how compliance impacted the effectiveness of the lockdown.[19] Were there factors such as the movement of migrants during the lockdown that contributed to the diffusion of the virus across India? It is certainly plausible, but at the time of writing there were no definitive epidemiological studies that had addressed this question.

In a final assessment, we must also must keep in mind that much more was known about the virus, how it is transmitted, how deadly it is and how best to treat the disease at the end of 2020 than was known at the time of the lockdown in March. We can retrospectively judge the decision, but in March, the true extent of susceptibility and transmission was not known. Even in October when European countries implemented 'second lockdowns' they did so in a targeted manner, learning from their past experiences and reviewing newly acquired information on how the virus was spread.

All said and done, we will be assessing the monumental impact of India's lockdown for years.

# 19

# Endgame

How will the pandemic end?

The SARS-CoV-2 pandemic will formally end when the herd immunity threshold is reached, and an average infection can no longer reproduce itself. Just as the WHO is the official body that declares a pandemic, it will be the one that will decide when it is over. But a pandemic ending and a virus getting eradicated are two different things. SARS-CoV-2 will continue to infect people. This virus isn't going anywhere soon.

A threat to maintaining herd immunity is the birth of new children who are susceptible and the loss of immunity among those who have been infected. Millions of children are born each year without immunity acquired from infection. Among those who are infected, the duration and durability of immunity are currently unknown. That said, those who have been infected once are expected to have some level of protective immunity.

On the other hand, some people may not be fully susceptible even though they've never been infected. Children under the age of ten, for example, seem less susceptible to infection. There's a theory that past infection with other viruses offers some partial immunity, possibly through immune memory. This is an exciting line of inquiry.

A lot of what happens immediately after the pandemic depends on the durability of immunity. A study which modelled SARS-CoV-2 transmission on parameters determined for two circulating human coronaviruses predicted that in the absence of lifelong immunity, the virus may enter permanent circulation.[1] If immunity either from a vaccine or from infection isn't lifelong, it's likely that later infections may be less severe than the first one, because people will have partial immunity. But even after the pandemic appears to die out, the virus may cause flare-ups from time to time.

New influenza subtypes that cause pandemics also transform into less deadly variants over time; that explains why there are fewer people who are completely susceptible in a population after a pandemic ends. This is akin to the immunity from flu vaccines, even when protection isn't perfect. The resulting flu is milder. And with mutations that allow the virus to evade the immune system and infect cells, there may be seasonal SARS-CoV-2 just as there are seasonal flu and common cold infections.

Since they are viruses that also cause acute respiratory infections, pandemic subtypes of influenza serve as a conceptual model for what we might expect for SARS-CoV-2. When pandemic influenza spills over from an animal and infects people, it may result in a more severe disease, especially if it is a subtype that's never been seen in people before. Pandemic influenza virus goes around infecting a lot of people who may get sick. This can happen quickly or over a few years.

After the first wave, there are subsequent waves, and then eventually the virus becomes endemic, circulating and ousting existing seasonal variants of influenza. Waves are cyclical patterns of infections in populations. A scenario can be imagined for SARS-CoV-2, in which after three waves of infections, the virus may become endemic in humans.[2] But with SARS-CoV-2, so far there has been no clear waxing and waning of infections typically seen with influenza. The virus did not go away in the summer of 2020, contrary to many early pronouncements.

We speak of the coming of waves, using terminology borrowed from influenza. However, many believe that this pandemic will be different. Waves disperse without human involvement, but coronavirus infections have not abated. 'I don't see this as a wave anymore. Waves are outdated. We have peaks and valleys,' said Michael Osterholm, a prominent infectious diseases researcher.[3]

It is likely that vaccines will not offer durable sterilizing immunity, or in other words, there may be no lifelong prevention of SARS-CoV-2 infections even with vaccination. However, this is also the case with seasonal flu vaccines which have to be taken every year. A vaccine that lessens symptomatic disease or severity might reduce mortality in a few years as opposed to decades. But it is likely that many people will not take a vaccine even when it is widely available. That would pose a significant challenge for reaching the herd immunity threshold.

Only two diseases have been completely eradicated in history: smallpox in humans and rinderpest in cows. A third disease, SARS, subsided, but its causative virus may remain in animal reservoirs. Reservoir animals pose a challenge for the eradication of diseases. There are many examples of reservoir animals causing a resurgence in infectious diseases. Humans gave armadillos leprosy and now infections in people periodically arise again from contact with armadillos. Even if we were to wipe out leprosy from humans, it would remain in armadillos. Similarly, eliminating SARS-CoV-2 from human populations may not eradicate the virus altogether, as it may live on in reservoirs in other susceptible animals. From these reservoir animals—minks, ferrets and cats—the virus might reinfect humans.

In contrast to viruses such as influenza and coronaviruses that cause acute respiratory infections, those that cause chronic infections often simply shift from one country to another. They can serve as an alternate model for what might be expected after the COVID-19 pandemic ends. The end of a pandemic may not equate with the end of localized spread. There may continue to be significant hotspots of disease and infection for years to come. HIV/AIDS still rages on in parts of Africa, though the rate of transmission is no longer what it used to be in many other parts of the world.

In the early days of microbiology, it was thought that germs that cause infectious diseases evolve inside hosts to become less detrimental over time. This was conventional wisdom for many years, but since then it has been shown that there are trade-offs to infection. Viruses grow inside hosts in order to spread. In this process, they use up host resources, destroy cells and tissues, and fight against immune resources. This causes disease. From our point-of-view as host, disease is what we worry about the most. In fact, disease is an inevitable cost to spreading.

There is an enticing theory that one of the coronaviruses that circulate in humans and cause common colds, OC43, was also responsible for a very poorly studied pandemic in 1889.[4] It has been speculated that this coronavirus jumped from cows into humans and then infected a lot of people, after which time it became less deadly.

If a virus evolves into a mutant that creates a lot of copies of itself, but in the process kills off its host or provokes a strong immune response from a host that clears it very quickly, it won't be able to spread efficiently. If on the other hand, the virus is slow in replicating and an infected person doesn't infect more than one additional person, it fades from the population. Neither is optimal for the spread of a virus. From the parasite's 'perspective', an ideal middle ground might be one in which it is neither a pushover nor a fast and efficient killer. Often, in the balance, there is an arms race between the immunity of the host and the infectivity of the virus.

Right now, SARS-CoV-2 is spreading quite efficiently and rapidly within human populations because we are susceptible to infection. Over time, the dynamics of transmission will change in ways that are difficult to predict.

Ultimately, when people ask when the pandemic will be over, they are not simply interested in biological reduction in infections, they want to know when life will return to the way it was in pre-pandemic times. And there are no orderly processes that can turn back the clock to the prior social and economic order. We must wait and observe what becomes the new normal.

# 20

# Impact

'Each man's death diminishes me,
For I am involved in mankind.
Therefore, send not to know
For whom the bell tolls,
It tolls for thee'

—John Donne,
'For Whom the Bell Tolls'

It is difficult to grasp the scale of the pandemic on human lives while we continue to live through it. Every day we are struck by headlines about disease, death and destruction that will haunt us for decades. Many of us have been infected, and it is quite possible that we know people who did not recover. Still, looking beyond the headlines to the many other ways in which the world abruptly changed is warranted, even if it provides only a fraction of the stories that blip on our radars.

Take, for example, sports. The impact of the pandemic was swift, with many leagues calling off matches. The 2020 Olympics which were originally slated to start in Tokyo in July were postponed to 2021. The UEFA Euro 2020 tournament was also put off until 2021. The thirteenth edition of the Indian Premier

League was postponed in March; it started in the United Arab Emirates in September with matches played in the absence of fans in stadiums.

The pandemic impacted lives in other ways as well. Overall violent crimes fell during the early 2020 lockdowns because criminals had fewer opportunities to interact with their potential victims who were more likely to be isolated in their own homes. However, there were exceptions. Taking advantage of the closure due to the pandemic, thieves stole a painting by celebrated Dutch master Vincent Van Gogh from a museum outside Amsterdam. The museum announced the theft on 30 March, which, in a cruel twist of fate, is the painter's birthday.

As facemasks became more prevalent in stopping disease, they also clouded identity. Some criminals used them for nefarious means. For example, in May, an imprisoned man in Chicago escaped by wearing a facemask and assuming the identity of another inmate who was supposed to be released.

The world was not prepared for social distancing. In April, a woman in New York City who did not maintain appropriate distance from others was arrested and held with two dozen other women for two days. After returning, she had to self-isolate. To maintain an appropriate distance, a Christian priest used a toy water-gun to squirt holy water at parishioners in Michigan. Other services for churches, mosques and temples were conducted by videoconference.

During the early 2020 lockdowns, rivers became cleaner and bluer skies were observed, all as a result of the cessation of human activities. With few cars on the roads, few factories running and limited farming activities in neighbouring states, the skies of Delhi became pollution free in April. It was possible to see the Himalayas from Chandigarh. The canals of Venice were clear. Air quality improved due to stalling of factory, automotive and agricultural practices. Global emissions for 2020 were predicted to drop by as much as 7 per cent, the greatest such drop since World War II.

Filming of shows and movies stopped abruptly, and slowly restarted towards the end of 2020. With theatres closed, some movies were released directly to streaming platforms. With limited new content and large audiences at home, channels began to telecast 'reruns'. Once the lockdown was over in India, TV serials began shooting with appropriate distancing. COVID-19 began to be inserted into storylines as plot-twists.

When the world does not show up for work, unique situations arise. In April, in the United States, two million chickens had to be killed and destroyed because due to work-at-home orders there was no one to slaughter them for the poultry industry.[1]

Animals took over the streets in many cities, but we also noticed animals more from our balconies and windows. In May, a gang of monkeys in Meerut attacked a medical laboratory technician and fled with blood samples of four patients who had tested positive and were undergoing treatment.[2] A Bolivian orchestra was stuck in a castle in Germany surrounded by forests with twenty-three known packs of wolves.

For all the criticisms of human society, in many ways the earth did come together on an unprecedented scale to face a new challenge. Many people did stay indoors. They wore masks for each other. Exhausted hospital workers were greeted by nightly ovations from balconies and windows. Some proprietors instituted rent freezes, employers paid workers in advance and private citizens set up kitchens with free meals and helped migrants to return home.

## On society

As humans we have a distinct advantage over the virus. We know how it spreads and can adapt our behaviour accordingly. The virus is hardwired to act in one way. It will continue to infect exactly in that same manner. But in order to defeat the virus, we also must *want* to adapt.

The biological complexities of the virus will be understood sooner than the social complexities of people. We can calculate the affinity of the SARS-CoV-2 spike to the ACE2 receptor and how much greater it is than that of the spike of SARS coronavirus. But how can someone who lives in crowded slums physically distance or quarantine? How can someone who has no access to water or soap wash their hands as frequently as advised?

There's the biology of the virus and how it affects different populations: severity according to age, and other diseases and conditions. And that is only the 'envelope' of the social virus. Jutting out like spikes are race, class, access to healthcare and gender. Biology will not solve the lack of social safety. Nor will it usher racial equality.

The fact is that there was a hierarchy of misery. SARS-CoV-2 did not affect everyone equally. There are those who were biologically vulnerable because of age or underlying conditions. And there are those who were socially vulnerable through greater exposure, malnutrition, poverty and lack of access to healthcare facilities.

It is true that viruses know no borders, but they are carried by people. Communities in Asia, Latin America and parts of Africa are separated by economic wealth, even though they are often right next to each other. In India, Brazil, Mexico and Chile affluent travellers and expatriates first brought the virus to their home countries from travel abroad. Then, the virus spread from wealthier neighbourhoods to poorer ones with fewer services, often through domestic workers. For example, by mid-June people living in poorer neighbourhoods in São Paulo were ten times more likely to die than those in affluent ones.

Minorities developed COVID-19 infection more frequently and succumbed to disease at alarming rates.[3] Blacks and Hispanics were disproportionately affected in the United States, the country worst hit by the pandemic in 2020. Racial minorities suffer disproportionately from known conditions that cause more severe outcomes such as heart disease, diabetes and obesity. But concerns went beyond these medical conditions. Blacks and Latinos were more than three times as likely to be infected and twice as likely to die from COVID-19. Social factors determined outcomes.

There was a vicious cycle that was only further laid bare by the pandemic. Racial minorities are poor and live in settings that are crowded, urban and with less access to top-notch healthcare facilities.[4] Many of them are 'essential workers'. So, in addition to medical conditions, and disparities with healthcare, they were required to go in harm's way.

In the United States, Brazil, India and many other countries race, religion and nationality indicate where people live, and type of housing and neighbourhoods have a direct correlation to services available. High housing density, low access to education, low security, crime and risky jobs especially in urban areas are problematic. Life expectancies vary in these large, heterogeneous nations.

Outbreaks occurred in migrant dormitories in Singapore, a country that had been initially lauded for its handling of the pandemic. There were similar outbreaks in Dubai, where many economic migrants also lived. Major outbreaks in the United States and in Germany occurred in meatpacking plants.[5] In the US, many Hispanics worked in these plants.

It was easy for people in positions of social and economic privilege to weather out the adverse effects of the lockdown, and to say that such measures needed to continue indefinitely until we felt safe to go outside. But what was there to offer in terms of advice to the person who had nowhere to distance? There was the tragedy of those dying of exhaustion, without food, without water, run over by trains and because they could not get cyclone relief. There was also the tragedy of those forced to walk to death or die infected in a prison cell or deported across borders.

Low socioeconomic status alone is a risk factor for death independent of other risk factors. Being able to work from home, participate in social events remotely and maintain a modicum of a normal life is a privilege. To the disadvantaged, these are not simply available. How, for example, is an autowallah to work from home? Poor people are also less likely to have access to good healthcare, knowledge of risks and how the disease is spread, and insurance. Consequently, they are less likely to also seek help for symptoms.

Many systemic and structural injustices are based on differences in community, caste, tribe, religion, wealth and appearance. During the Black Death there was mass persecution of Jews in Europe. Families were burned alive. HIV/AIDS led to persecution of homosexuals and drug users. Both after SARS and after COVID-19 there was a victimization of Chinese and Asian populations and those who look East Asian in the eyes of the attackers, regardless of ethnicity or nationality.

Women were disproportionately impacted during the pandemic. Women constitute around 70 per cent of healthcare and social workers around the world. These professions are at the frontlines of the pandemic. Women also represent 70 per cent of the world's poor. But economic strain is not the only aspect. In addition, childcare, household duties and caring for the elderly and sick routinely fall on women. These responsibilities are not only activities that take time, but the mental effort of planning. Women are the first to be expected to become teachers of children and nurses of the elderly at home and put their careers and financial freedom on hold.

Distancing is about cutting ourselves off from society for a time physically to slow down the spread of disease. It is not about cutting ourselves off from society mentally. All of us who are privileged must think harder about the disadvantaged. Everyone suffers, but it is always the vulnerable who suffer the most and for the longest duration. And this is one aspect of the pandemic we must pause to think about. People who spread the disease are our neighbours, our colleagues, our relatives and our children.

## On public health

The impact of the virus, beyond direct concerns of disease resulting from it, has been swift and severe. Measures implemented during the pandemic may have serious effects on broader long-term public health. Alarmingly, the number of hospital visits for those with serious conditions has declined globally, perhaps out of concern of getting infected with SARS-CoV-2 during visitations. As a result, chronic cancer, heart disease or diabetes patients are seeking medical care less frequently than before the pandemic.

A telemedicine approach using available technology, including consultations via phone and text messaging, was used for doctors' appointments. Unfortunately, vaccinations cannot be done without visits. Childhood vaccination is an area of particular concern, since many parents are simply opting to defer or avoid getting their children vaccinated for certain infectious diseases altogether.

Since volunteers are unable to administer polio vaccines, an unfortunate rise in polio in the last remaining pockets of this eradicable disease is expected. Due to lack of protection from vaccination, millions of children may be at risk for measles. The year 2020 was predicted to be the first one with a significant rise in child mortality in decades.

Prenatal and postnatal care, especially in the developing world was also disrupted. Many simply decided to forego having children altogether during the pandemic. Adoptions were also down: a sign that people were putting off thinking about expanding their families.

The pandemic heightened the disparity between the Global North and South. Countries as distant as Ecuador and South Africa faced a shortage of test kits that forced them to hold off on testing, a key step in controlling COVID-19. On the other hand, among the privileged in Western countries, there was a heightened demand for plastic surgery: many affluent people simply did not like how they looked in online meetings.

## On mental health

The drawing of white circles on roads to maintain appropriate distancing was a poignant visual reminder that John Donne was wrong: during a pandemic, everyone *is* an island. Seasons change while we stay indoors. Flowers blossom in our absence.

The pandemic presented several immediate causes of stress: loss of livelihood, potential sickness and death, and uncertainty. The lockdowns instituted globally increased alcohol consumption and abuse, isolation and anxiety. The support systems of extended friends and families available to migratory populations and nuclear families were extinguished.

While loneliness is a subjective perception, over a period of time it can lead to depression, anxiety, cognitive decline, difficulty falling and staying asleep, and increase in blood pressure. Loneliness can make anyone more prone to adverse health conditions, but the elderly and poor are especially vulnerable. The elderly in particular suffered not only the worst effects of COVID-19 in nursing homes and eldercare facilities common in many industrialized countries, but also curtailed visits from children and grandchildren. The anxiety of dying alone is real. And there is a horrible incompleteness in not being able to share the last moments of life.

Friends and family were unable to see loved ones who were hospitalized. Families were torn apart by restrictions on travel and immigration suspensions. Those who lost loved ones were unable to see them in their last moments.

Those who did not face loneliness or isolation were also troubled. Immense mental burden was caused from repeated exposure to thoughts of hopelessness and uncertainty. Losing one's source of income caused anxiety, and this was magnified in disadvantaged sections of society. Compounding the economic burden was the shame felt with joblessness.

Children are a vulnerable population. In addition to loss of family income, with the loss of regular meals, widespread malnutrition is predicted. Three hundred million children who relied on midday meals in schools faced hunger. The impact on growth might affect an entire generation. Children lost a chance to interact and classes were disrupted from nursery to postgraduate levels. In addition, in many countries, child abuse at home is primarily detected in school: when schools were closed, more children were put at risk.

COVID-19 and domestic violence have been referred to as 'twin public health emergencies'. This assertion comes from the understanding that not everyone is safe at home. In the absence of public scrutiny and in close quarters, abusers can resort to domestic violence with impunity. The abuse many children and adults faced is expected to have long-term physical and psychological effects.

Social interactions are believed to play a significant role in suicide prevention. Thoughts of helplessness and self-harm are exacerbated in extended periods of social isolation. Close contacts who might have otherwise routinely checked on those with depression and clinical anxiety were shut out during this time, and this disconnection might ultimately increase suicide risk. It has been reported that suicides increased during the 1918-19 H1N1 influenza pandemic in the United States and among the elderly in Hong Kong during the 2003 SARS epidemic. A true reckoning of the mental toll of the pandemic will take decades.

Humans are social animals. Experts warned that long after the viral pandemic has subsided, we might have to contend with a 'mental health pandemic'. What will be the outcome of loss of livelihood or sedentary, work-from-home lifestyles? What will be the effect of a sudden transition to isolation and distancing? There are no easy and immediate answers to these questions.

## On the economy

With sustained global growth for many years since the Great Recession, global equities at all-time highs and unemployment rates at lows in many countries, it is natural to pine for the halcyon days of 2019. The rude shock of 2020 is that the pillars of the global economy were ill prepared for a sustained pandemic. By the end of 2020, world trade was expected to fall 13.4 per cent, the steepest decline in my own lifetime. Globally, foreign direct investment was expected to fall by 20 per cent or more.

Job losses were swift and severe with hundreds of millions of livelihoods impacted, and predictions that a recovery might take decades. Poverty and starvation due to job losses and lack of opportunities threatened to stunt an entire generation of vulnerable populations. Around 2 billion people, most of them in low-income and low-middle income brackets, earn their living in the informal economy. With the loss of livelihood, starvation is an immediate concern.

The socioeconomic inequalities in every country were heightened during the first lockdown phase of the pandemic. Who can work from home? Clearly, not everyone. Those in the service sector and in management, technology, finance and business were able to shift to online and Internet-based platforms while those in industries such as manufacturing and construction were not.

Those who have less education, immigrants, racial minorities and women were often the quickest to lose their jobs. On the other hand, jobs in public transport, retail, health and social care were deemed essential, but along with the 'essential' badge came greater potential exposure.

Workers in the much-vaunted 'gig economy' who drove cars hailed by ride-sharing apps and delivered food and other goods on demand had to weigh the risk of getting sick against the risk of running out of money. As co-workers fell ill, transportation workers and those in meatpacking plants were expected to continue working. One said poignantly, 'We don't get paid enough to risk our life.'

Remittances from temporary workers, which sustained many families and formed a substantial part of the gross domestic product of many countries, fell. In some countries, undocumented workers who were potentially infected were deported without treatment. Anti-immigrant sentiment spiked in many countries that were hit especially hard, especially as job losses accelerated. Often, those who looked different were targeted.

During the first lockdowns of 2020, global supply chains that ran through China and India were disrupted. Countries and communities began to jostle with one another for exclusive access to essential drugs, facemasks and mechanical ventilators. Countries engaged in bidding wars against one another, politicians called on personal favours and suppliers diverted shipments at the last minute. The first few weeks of March were a free-for-all. Factories across the world retooled to manufacture personal protective and medical equipment.

Consumer confidence plummeted. People spent more money on groceries, news and online streaming content, and less on travel, dining and fashion. Clothing, jewellery and accessories are usually bought in person after touch and trial. These purchases were put on hold. The purchase of cosmetics and personal care supplies declined globally since people were not going out. Many fashion brands decided to make masks.

Many industries went into freefall because of restrictions on movement. For example, with ships idled, the seafood industry sank. Stocks of certain commercially important fish increased marginally, but consumer prices also rose. There was a shortage of many goods, often because there were no workers to tend to animals, harvest crops or work in factories. Suppliers of food and sanitation products in bulk to restaurants and hotels suddenly found that they needed new distribution systems and sizes for individual retail consumers.

In Western countries, irate shoppers fought over overpriced and understocked rolls of toilet paper. In fact, in a sign of the times, many people took photos of empty supermarket shelves and shared them on social media. The price at which crude oil was traded fell below $0.00 in April while the price of edible commodities like rice rose to seven-year highs.[6]

Schools and universities closed in-person classes, and some went to online-only formats. Teachers mulled over how to design course curricula for distance learning. Parents had to decide if they would send their children to schools when they opened. The pandemic disrupted fieldwork and teaching, with many institutions only allowing coronavirus-related research to continue. In the meantime, numerous researchers from disparate fields pivoted to coronavirus research.

Transportation, especially for discretionary purposes, was curtailed severely. Tourism ground to a halt. Once busy hotels in cities such as Paris, Barcelona and Venice suddenly found that they were vacant. Cafes and restaurants shuttered. When they reopened, they were often forced to cater to delivery and takeout-only options. Cruise ships and airlines which were particularly badly hit cancelled entire routes, often stranding their crews at sea. It was not clear how many businesses would be able to remain viable as they burned through enormous amounts of cash.

There had already been massive damage to businesses that require humans in proximity and events that required people all together at once—sports, conferences and recreational travel. How and when will these businesses recover? For discretionary travel and events, it is too early to say. First, health concerns will need to be addressed to assure that it is safe to enjoy these activities again. But second, and arguably, equally important is the need to address the crisis in confidence. Many of the industries, small businesses, family-owned shops and restaurants are simply not coming back to life.

## On technology

SARS was the first new virus for which information was available in real time. In 2009, H1N1 influenza was the first pandemic of the social media age (though it hardly made a splash in popular social networks). COVID-19 is the first work-from-home pandemic.

The most immediate change in the lives of those who had to get accustomed to working or learning from home was the complete reliance on the Internet. This created not only a chasm between those whose jobs, mainly in the services sector, could shift to home environments and those whose couldn't. It created a rift between those who had reliable broadband access and those who didn't. According to a study, India ranked as the least-prepared out of forty-two countries analysed with respect to a work-from-a-distance infrastructure.[7]

Before the Industrial Revolution, jobs were broadly defined by output, as opposed to fixed times. Later, time spent onsite became important. We might see a shift to middle ground. With more work-from-home options available in the knowledge-based economy and certain high-skilled and high-paying jobs likely to become permanently available to employees working from home, there might be downstream effects on other jobs. Offices, especially in large cities, were costly to maintain, but they supported not only those who worked in them, but also those who performed ancillary functions. Working from home or from satellite offices connected by technology became necessary due to the pandemic, but many workers might not return once it is over.

Over time, online meetings became the norm and globally chatter over lighting for meetings, virtual backgrounds and appropriate books to keep in bookshelves behind became hot topics on social media. Real life spilled over on to work; spouses, children and pets occupied the same space and time, creating pressure, and no boundaries between home and work. School and college went completely online, and brought challenges of managing classrooms, setting goals and grading homework.

Television shows, especially those with hosts interviewing guests, went online. Live audiences were gone. The cinematic possibilities of videoconferencing platforms were explored. Some television shows were filmed with actors speaking their lines from their own homes. Museums and arts groups began virtual displays of collections. There were online book readings, stand-up comedy routines and music recitals. Sports events were held in empty stadiums.

Technology also made contact-tracing and health-tracking applications available on smartphones. Singapore, China, Taiwan, Israel and South Korea all used geolocation data from cell phones for sending instant alerts and digital contact tracing, but there were concerns regarding security and privacy when tracking a massive number of citizens.

# 21

# Aftermath

'Everyone knows that pestilences have a way of recurring in the world; yet somehow, we find it hard to believe in ones that crash down on our heads from a blue sky'

—Albert Camus, *La Peste*

Scientists had been predicting a major pandemic for at least thirty years with a remarkable degree of clarity and with what seems like foresight now. SARS-CoV-2 caused havoc because there was a mix of factors both in the biological makeup of the virus and in the way that it spread early on. Humans might not have been responsible for its origin, but we were responsible for its spread.

Alarmingly, there have been many new and re-emerging diseases that have cropped up as global threats over the last two decades. These diseases such as SARS, Ebola, MERS, Zika, H1N1 and Nipah caused tragic losses of life but never rose to the scale of destruction of SARS-CoV-2. Part of that was certainly due to prompt human intervention, but part of it was also due to *luck*—all these viruses had flaws in the way that they were transmitted compared to SARS-CoV-2. In hindsight, one of the early precipitating factors is that SARS-CoV-2 was first detected in Wuhan, a city larger than New York or London, instead of in a remote village where it might have died out after a minor outbreak.

But globally our response was also uneven. Even as late as January when the virus was ravaging through China, there was a sense of calm elsewhere. Were we collectively in denial? Were we thinking that this can't really be *that* bad? That this can't happen to *us*?

After the pandemic ends, there will be a push to fund major efforts to study and control infectious diseases. We can't know exactly how or when the next pandemic will strike, but we can predict the broad nature of future threats. After all, the best time to prepare for the next pandemic is when you are in one.

The key drivers of the emergence of disease-causing organisms are not expected to change in the near future and in many cases may be accelerating. New infectious diseases come from animals in close proximity to people. High population density, mixed agriculture, the presence of live markets where exotic animals are butchered and sold, and living quarters close to animals served as an incubator for the transfer of SARS coronavirus in 2002 and SARS-CoV-2 in 2019. These are the same precipitating factors for the periodic emergence of avian and swine flu. Surveillance is difficult because the symptoms of respiratory diseases are similar, but early identification and isolation of cases are essential to stop the spread once a disease emerges.

Loss of biodiversity and changes in land use are major drivers of pandemics. Species that adapt to interactions with humans will become a source of new infections. Unsustainable exploitation of the environment changes interactions between people and animals. It is estimated that more than 30 per cent of new diseases identified since 1960 have been caused by changes in land use.[1]

Climate change is a major challenge for humanity that will impact all aspects of our life and will also cause an increase in insect-vector-borne diseases.[2] With climate change there will be shifts in the distribution of insects that will expose more people to deadly diseases. Mild winters will also change the lifecycles of vectors so that diseases develop much earlier. In addition, climate change will cause the movement of people and animals that will accelerate the spread of existing diseases and exposure to new ones. Small temperature increases can greatly affect transmission potential. The emergence of tick-borne encephalitis in Scandinavia has been tied to climate change. Globally, temperature increases of around 2°C would increase the number of people at risk of malaria by 3-5 per cent or several hundred million people.

What will be the nature of the infectious disease that will strike us next? Since these are the last few pages, I will throw caution to the wind and speculate on the nature of the next infectious agent that may cause a pandemic.

The next pandemic may be caused by a virus that jumps from an animal into people. Since we will never have seen it before, we will not have acquired immunity. Viruses that have jumped from animal reservoirs and have caused outbreaks in people include rabies, Hendra and West Nile Virus. These, however, do not transmit efficiently in humans.

Almost all infectious diseases identified in the last three decades are caused by RNA viruses. RNA viruses are also the cause of all the major pandemics that have occurred in the last century. Therefore, it is safe to assume that this class of viruses will continue to be a threat.

Other viral diseases that are not likely to become pandemics include Nipah and MERS: they are exceptionally lethal, but they do not transmit well among people. They are responsible for one or a few chains of human-to-human transmission, but outbreaks end after that. If the viruses that cause these infections were to mutate to be able to transmit efficiently, we would have a serious problem. More likely, a pandemic will be caused by species jump followed by efficient human-to-human transmission as we've observed for HIV/AIDS, Ebola, SARS, COVID-19 and new strains of pandemic influenza.

But transmission alone doesn't define a pandemic. Its deadliness is what makes us take note. In 2009 a new H1N1 strain spread across the world, yet many people were unaware that the WHO had declared it a pandemic. They may have been infected and may simply have brushed it off. The reason H1N1 in 2009 did not receive the same interest or warrant the same measures as the H1N1 strain of 1918 is that it was not as deadly.

How a virus spreads determines its pandemic potential also. Acute respiratory infectious diseases like COVID-19 and influenza cause severe pandemics.[3] Their quick spread means that a large population may be infected before measures are in place. The time course of an infection is rapid; for influenza it proceeds in days; for COVID-19 it is longer, but still in weeks. Only a few people may be symptomatic, causing greater difficulty in identifying silent infections in a period when people are infectious. These two factors combined make travel bans and restrictions less effective than for slower infections spread by other means. Air travel by asymptomatic or pre-symptomatically infected people was a major contributor to the rapid spread of SARS and COVID-19.

It is quite possible that the next pandemic may also be caused by another respiratory virus. These viruses are the greatest threats because of how they spread. It is easier to isolate someone with a disease that causes problems in the gastrointestinal tract such as vomiting or diarrhoea. We can choose to drink different water or eat different food, but we must all breathe the same air.

Even for a devastating sexually transmitted disease like HIV/AIDS that has caused tens of millions of deaths, how it spreads limits its ability to spread rapidly. This isn't meant to downplay the significant health burden of HIV/AIDS, only to highlight features of respiratory viruses that confer pandemic potential.

A pandemic can originate anywhere but there are certain drivers that make more regions more likely than others. Many of the drivers converge in a few hotspots for the emergence of viruses with pandemic potential.

In parts of South and East Asia, influenza virus subtypes occur year-round in many types of poultry, but especially in ducks. Avian influenza strains are usually very lethal in people, but do not usually spread well. But both human and avian influenza subtypes can infect pigs, which are 'mixing vessels' for influenza. In pigs, avian influenza strains undergo wholesale genetic alterations with other influenza strains that allow them to infect people better.

There are many distinct types of influenza virus that circulate in animals, but very few new viruses cross over into humans. Of those that do, fewer still transmit from one human to another effectively. We know the reason for this is what we'd expect for all viruses: the new virus isn't quite adept at picking the lock of the human receptor. But due to the ability to mix and match pieces from different subtypes to create new viruses that can break into human cells well while evading immune response, it is only a matter of time before a subtype of influenza causes another pandemic.

Two viruses that worry scientists right now are H1N1 and H3N2, which are related to viruses that caused earlier pandemics. But that's not all we have to worry about. Avian influenza, also known as bird flu, might cause the most severe issues if it became transmissible. H5N1 is overly concerning since it has a very high mortality rate. As I mentioned earlier, avian influenza doesn't transmit very effectively in humans, but this strain is very lethal. This has extremely high pandemic potential.

Just like the H1N1 virus that caused the worst influenza pandemic in history, H5N1 is an avian virus. H5N1 was first spotted in geese in China in 1996. The following year it was detected in people during an outbreak in poultry in Hong Kong. That was the first big global bird flu scare. And six countries have poultry that are known to harbour the H5N1 virus. Along with China, Bangladesh, Indonesia, Vietnam and Egypt, India is one of them.

So far, we've been exceptionally lucky that this lethal virus doesn't have the ability to transmit effectively in humans.

Otherwise, a pandemic of catastrophic proportions would be on the cards. Approximately 60 per cent of those infected by this virus have died.

H7N9 is another influenza subtype that we have to worry about. It first spread from birds to people in 2013. Since then, it has infected people in five waves, killing 40 per cent of them. Fortunately, it too doesn't spread well among people.

We can expect with an extremely high degree of certainty that influenza pandemics will continue to plague humans in the future. The ingredients of an influenza pandemic are all in place and it's only a matter of time before the next one strikes.

A majority of the diseases that have emerged in the last fifty years have come from wildlife. Some of these like Ebola pass directly to us through hunting of wildlife and growing and selling of exotic animals. Others like new strains of influenza pass from wildlife to people through infected livestock.

The cost of this pandemic will be enormous. What will be the cost of the next one? Preventing the emergence of infectious diseases and pandemics will require a paradigm shift in thinking. We will need to integrate costs of the next pandemic into production and consumption. Disease risk assessment will need to be integrated into public policy and development projects. We must proactively invest in the development of a pipeline of drugs and vaccines before the next pandemic. Perhaps an equivalent of the Paris Agreement on climate change will be necessary for international cooperation on emerging infectious diseases.

The world must work together to stop the SARS-CoV-2 pandemic. When the next pandemic strikes, we must be better prepared for it.

# 22

# Future

'No matter how selfish our motives, we can no longer be indifferent to the suffering of others. The microbe that felled one child in a distant continent yesterday can reach yours today and seed a global pandemic tomorrow.' These words were written by the Nobel Prize-winning microbiologist Joshua Lederberg in 1988.[1] Yet, they ring equally true today.

Infectious diseases loom large in the life of anyone who has spent time in the developing world. Measures are taken every day to avoid bad water and vectors. Prior to the pandemic, when was the last time the Western industrialized world was gripped by a pervasive threat of an infectious disease? Over a century, the wealthier nations of the world improved their access to clean and healthy food. There is a relationship between geography and the shadow of diseases, between socioeconomic status and treatment standards, between poverty and access to medicine for curable diseases.

Cholera largely disappeared from the United States over a century ago. And yet it is a life-threatening problem elsewhere. HIV/AIDS no longer gets the same headlines globally because it disproportionately impacts sub-Saharan Africa. Ebola ravaged Western Africa for years, remaining in the mind of most elsewhere a distant problem associated with poor African villages. Most are blissfully unaware that had it not been contained in Lagos in 2014, it could've been a much bigger tragedy than it was.

According to the WHO, three of the top ten global killers are infectious diseases. The WHO has also estimated that acute respiratory infections cause 4 million deaths each year of which nearly half are in children.

Take, for example, TB. A quarter of the world's people might be infected by *Mycobacterium tuberculosis*, the causative agent of TB. Roughly 10 million people around the world fall ill from this disease each year. Over a million die.

Well-heeled global citizens everywhere can tell you all the features of the latest smartphone within minutes of launch, they can tell you the storyline of a superhero movie on the Friday that it releases globally. Meanwhile for years we are collectively unaware of threats of looming infectious diseases.

Many of the regions that responded relatively well to the first onslaught of the pandemic had prior experience in dealing with outbreaks of infectious diseases. The populations took risks seriously, leaders knew whom to turn to in the moment of crisis, and strategies were based on established science. Public health was not pitted against the economy; rather it was considered a prerequisite for the functioning of the economy. The strategies in South Korea, Hong Kong, Kerala and Rwanda were vastly different given the different structures of populations and local governments, but all had this in common.

In the early months of the pandemic, it can be argued that some countries that suffered from SARS over a decade ago learned a lesson, while others that didn't failed to initially take the virus seriously. Countries that faced SARS were ready this time.

Travelling though East Asia even before the pandemic, I noticed people wearing facemasks. It is culturally acceptable. If you are sick with a respiratory disease, it is expected that you wear one. In many countries, you can walk into a convenience store and get an N95 respirator. The discomfort is tolerated. Wearing a facemask is a preventive health measure, not an ideological statement.

The pandemic did not hit all countries equally at once. Countries that were impacted later could've learned from the expertise of others. For example, experts from China commented on the first lockdown in northern Italy to ensure that it was effective.

In January 2020, instead of using a perfectly reliable diagnostic test kit, the US CDC decided to develop a new kit which did not work. Contaminations meant that for nearly two months, the scale of infections in the United States was not known, testing criteria had to be limited and infected people unknowingly spread the disease. This nightmare could have been averted had the CDC used the working kit that had already been developed.[2]

But the other aspect that needs to be examined involves complacency after the H1N1 influenza pandemic. In 2009, countries mounted a vast, costly exercise in response to a pandemic that did not have the serious consequences initially feared.[3] There is an interesting question that must be posed because preparation is done by humans and requires political, popular and human support. Did many countries underestimate this pandemic because they overestimated the last one?

## What happens next?

Envisioning what the future holds in store is like imagining what dry land is like while in a storm in the middle of the ocean. Even in the best of times, predicting the future is a risky enterprise. A devastating pandemic of this scale and severity imposes additional challenges because we have no reference point in the modern era for something like this. Off-the-cuff comments may be forgotten but writing tends to stick around and haunt the writer. If you're too certain with your pronouncements, you're almost certain to be wrong. If you're too vague, no one will read what you have to say.

We are only coming to terms with the direct fallout of the pandemic, but what will be the ramifications for long-term health and planning? What will be the implications for travel, for immigration and for commerce? Will countries continue to look inward once the pandemic is over?

Certain aspects of human life and society have changed due to the immediate effects of the pandemic. It is possible, therefore, to make short-term predictions. What will happen five, ten, or fifteen years down the road because of the ongoing, cataclysmic event and our responses to it are more difficult to say.

Will there be more public interest in interest in infectious diseases and medicine? Will it become a field that attracts more of the brightest minds as engineering, information technology, finance and business management have in preceding decades? Will physicians take up more active roles in framing public policy? Will economists stress-test catastrophic economic events of this nature?

Human societies are designed to maximize connections. Over the course of a day, most of us have dozens of close interactions with other people. The design of cities, buildings, jobs, transportation and commerce keeps the human need for connection in mind more than the rare threat of a disease that spreads by human-to-human interaction.

What can we say looking at the past? Based on a study of the H1N1 influenza pandemic of 1918, the historian Nancy Bristow writes, 'If history is any guide, not much will change in the wake of the COVID-19 pandemic.'[4] Yet, it is impossible to use history as guide, because the world has changed immensely in a century. In 1918, viruses had not been characterized. Colonial powers ruled the world and were in the middle of World War I. Commercial airline travel was non-existent. There was no Internet to allow the lay public to read research articles immediately and view daily statistics on illness and death.

In the United States, common drinking cups, which had previously been prevalent in schools and offices, were banned during the 1918 pandemic: they never staged a return. Will the pandemic of 2020 do the same for handshakes as many have predicted? Will more people in the world don facemasks at the first signs of a cough, as they have done in parts of Asia since the SARS outbreak seventeen years ago? Will more states in India invest in healthcare and build community-based surveillance systems, and learn as Kerala did after it successfully controlled the Nipah outbreak?

We can assume that the pandemic will irrevocably change some business practices. There will be more people working from home permanently and less business travel to meet clients and for conferences. Technological solutions that were embraced perhaps with a bit of trepidation during the pandemic will become wider habits.

Distancing is challenging in factories, warehouses, prisons, airplanes, dormitories and ships where space is maximized. Due to a premium being put on space in cities and the density of population, buildings have grown vertically. Property values have risen globally since the Great Recession. Gentrification had led to a return to economically disadvantaged areas. It is possible that there will be a reshaping of how urban spaces are used, with more people now moving outward instead of flocking to New York, Mumbai or London. But the experience of Hong Kong, Taiwan and Tokyo in the first year of the pandemic has demonstrated that even within densely populated cities, measures can be taken to keep infections low. There may be a reshaping of urban societies, but it is still too early to tell. People tend to go where there are economic opportunities.

More broadly, will humans finally address the pressing problems of the day which the pandemic brought into stark relief?

Problems of inequality, poor access to healthcare and economic opportunities, and lack of equal rights are prevalent globally.

The pandemic allows humans to face difficult challenges that we have been ignoring, instead of denying or downplaying them. It gives us a chance to reframe priorities and reimagine society.

As humans we tend to focus on *immediate* problems. Our ancestors were good at hiding from tigers and other dangerous animals, finding caves to sleep in when it was raining, and building a fire when it was cold. Longer-term planning for problems does not come easily. This is applicable to both people individually and to us as a species.

Countries faced with disparities that prevented adequate protection for all of their residents can choose to emerge with a reimagined and restructured society that is better prepared for future crises, or they can ignore the lessons of the pandemic and return to business as usual.

We are a vulnerable species and for all our control of the planet, we are subject to its vagaries. Climate change, the emergence and resurgence of infectious diseases, deforestation and the rapid loss of species, overconsumption and socioeconomic inequities can no longer be pushed under the carpet.

As far as the emergence of pandemics is concerned, all of these factors are inextricably linked. Climate change accelerates the emergence of new infectious diseases. Unsustainable exploitation of wildlife and natural resources puts people closer to reservoirs of new diseases.

I hope we all come out of this pandemic realizing that in a hot, crowded and interconnected world, we cannot afford to be parochial. If not for altruistic reasons, for selfish ones. A crisis that hits any part of the world or segment of society also affects us. Will we learn from the pandemic and prepare for other crises such as habitat destruction, climate change, the rise of antibiotic resistant diseases and the threat of nuclear war between belligerent states?

We keep asking ourselves, 'When will the pandemic end?' But we can't mark the end as the date when it is over only for those of us who are privileged. We know that the biological pandemic will end one day. What we must also ensure is that there is an end to the social one.

# Acknowledgements

I am grateful to everyone who made this book possible. First, and foremost, I must thank my family for their love and support, and for letting me focus on this book during weekends, in the evenings and late at night. They have had to sacrifice a lot, especially during my extended periods of mental distancing.

I thank my employers for paying the bills. They are not responsible for any opinions expressed here or any inaccuracies, both of which are solely my own.

One additional caveat is in order. This book does not purport to provide any medical advice. I am not a physician and am not qualified to diagnose anyone. If you feel that you are ill, you should seek professional help.

Any scientific writing becomes obsolete rapidly. Writing about a pandemic in the middle of one caused by a new virus is, therefore, fraught with peril. I have pored through thousands of articles and news stories over the past few months and have tried to ensure that the information presented here is accurate. However, over time, our understanding *will* change. This is inevitable. The expanding and self-correcting nature of science is beautiful and frustrating at the same time, and that is what compels many of us to be so enamoured by it. The physicist John Archibald Wheeler pointed out insightfully that we live on an island of knowledge surrounded by a sea of ignorance. As the island expands, the boundary between knowledge and ignorance also grows.

Thanks to Manasi Subramaniam of Penguin India for reaching out and discussing this project with me, and for giving me the freedom to run with it. Thanks to Shiny Das for her wonderful inputs. I am grateful to Kevin Davies, Krishna Ganesh, Ross Larue, Suvam Pal, Deblina Panigrahi, Sakshi Pandit and Parag Sahasrabudhe for the discussions. Thanks also to Siddharth Singh who first suggested that I write on this topic. I hope I have done justice to all those who put their faith in me.

I must also thank many people I do not know personally. I am grateful to the teachers who prepared lesson plans and taught children online, to the farmers who made sure we were all fed, to the first responders who kept civil society functioning, to the waste collectors and sanitation workers who kept other diseases from breaking out, to the public health officials who kept us informed through every public health emergency, to the artists and writers who provided much-needed creative and intellectual stimulus, to the scientists who helped us make sense of the unknown, and unquestionably, to the doctors and nurses who rose to the highest standards of their profession during this pandemic.

Lastly, I thank my many friends on social media, particularly on Twitter, whom I floated some of these ideas by (often unbeknownst to them). They know who they are: they are my extended family. *We'll get through this.*

# Notes

## Chapter 1: Parable

1. Wiersinga W.J., Rhodes A., Cheng A.C., Peacock S.J., Prescott H.C. 'Pathophysiology, transmission, diagnosis, and treatment of coronavirus disease 2019 (COVID-19): A Review'. *JAMA: Journal of the American Medical Association*. Published online 10 July 2020. doi:10.1001/jama.2020.12839

2. World Health Organization (WHO), 'Pneumonia of unknown cause: China'. Accessed 20 August 2020. https://www.who.int/csr/don/05-january-2020-pneumonia-of-unkown-cause-china/en/

3. 'India limits medicine exports after supplies hit by coronavirus'. World News. *Guardian*. Accessed 20 August 2020. https://www.theguardian.com/world/2020/mar/04/india-limits-medicine-exports-coronavirus-paracetamol-antibiotics

4. Helms J., Kremer S., Merdji H., et al. 'Neurologic features in severe SARS-COV-2 infection'. *New England Journal of Medicine*. 2020; 382 (23): 2268–270. doi:10.1056/NEJMc2008597

5. 'We cannot keep ignoring the possibility of airborne transmission. Here's how to address it'. *Washington Post*. Accessed 20 August 2020. https://www.washingtonpost.com/opinions/2020/05/26/key-stopping-covid-19-addressing-airborne-transmission/?hpid=hp_opinions-float-right-4-0_opinion-card-i-right%3Ahomepage%2Fstory-ans

6. 'Scientific papers on novel coronavirus doubling every 14 days'. Quartz. Published 8 April 2020. Accessed 16 August 2020. https://qz.com/1834521/scientific-papers-on-novel-coronavirus-doubling-every-14-days/

7. 'How a torrent of COVID science changed research publishing—in seven charts'. *Nature*. Published online 16 December 2020. https://www.nature.com/articles/d41586-020-03564-y

8. 'In the wake of the pandemic, life goes on in Wuhan, China'. *Washington Post*. Published 21 December 2020. https://www.washingtonpost.com/photography/2020/12/21/wuhan-goes-back-normal/

9. Claeson M., Hanson S. 'COVID-19 and the Swedish enigma.' *Lancet*. Published 22 December 2020. doi:https://doi.org/10.1016/S0140-6736(20)32750-1.

10. Islam N., Sharp S.J., Chowell G., et al. 'Physical distancing interventions and incidence of coronavirus disease 2019: Natural experiment in 149 countries'. *BMJ*. 2020; 370. doi:10.1136/bmj.m2743

11. 'Redefining vulnerability in the era of COVID-19'. *Lancet*. 2020; 395(10230): 1089. doi:10.1016/S0140-6736(20)30757-1

12. 'Covid in Europe: How countries are tackling second wave'. *Guardian*. Accessed 12 November 2020. https://www.theguardian.com/world/2020/oct/15/covid-in-europe-how-countries-are-tackling-second-wave

13. 'COVID-19: pandemic shatters more records in US, as states and cities tighten restrictions'. *New York Times*. Accessed 12 November 2020. https://www.nytimes.com/live/2020/11/12/world/covid-19-coronavirus-updates#the-us-again-broke-records-for-new-cases-more-than-160000-and-hospitalizations

14. Chang S., Pierson E., Koh P.W., et al. 'Mobility network models of COVID-19 explain inequities and inform reopening'. *Nature*. Published online 2020. doi:10.1038/s41586-020-2923-3

15. 'Implications of the emerging SARS-CoV-2 Variant VOC 202012/01'. Centers for Disease Control and Prevention. Published online 22 December 2020. https://www.cdc.gov/coronavirus/2019-ncov/more/scientific-brief-emerging-variant.html

16. Ibid.

17. Laxminarayan R., Wahl B., Dudala S.R., et al. 'Epidemiology and transmission dynamics of COVID-19 in two Indian states'. *Science*. Published online 30 September 2020. doi:10.1126/science.abd7672

18. 'Facial masking for Covid-19'. *New England Journal of Medicine*. Published online 23 October 2020. doi:10.1056/nejmc2030886; Gandhi M., Rutherford G.W. 'Facial masking for Covid-19: potential for "variolation" as we await a vaccine'. *New England Journal of Medicine*. 2020; 383(18): e101. doi:10.1056/nejmp2026913

19. Wiersinga W.J., Rhodes A., Cheng A.C., Peacock S.J., Prescott H.C. 'Pathophysiology, transmission, diagnosis, and treatment of coronavirus disease 2019 (COVID-19): a review'. *JAMA: Journal of the American Medical Association*. Published online 10 July 2020. doi:10.1001/jama.2020.12839

20. *Coronavirus Disease (COVID-19) Situation Report-183*. WHO. Published online 21 July 2020. https://www.who.int/docs/default-source/wha-70-and-phe/20200721-covid-19-sitrep-183.pdf

21. 'COVID-19 death rates are going down, and not just among the young and healthy'. *Health News: NPR*. Accessed 10 November 2020. https://www.npr.org/sections/health-shots/2020/10/20/925441975/studies-point-to-big-drop-in-covid-19-death-rates

22. Gilbert G.L. 'Commentary: SARS, MERS and COVID-19-new threats; old lessons'. *International Journal of Epidemiology*. 2020; 49(3): 726–28. doi:10.1093/ije/dyaa061

23. Zaki A.M., van Boheemen S., Bestebroer T.M., Osterhaus A.D.M.E., Fouchier R.A.M. 'Isolation of a novel coronavirus from a man with pneumonia in Saudi Arabia'. *New England Journal of Medicine*. 2012; 367(19): 1814–20. doi:10.1056/NEJMoa1211721

24. Donnelly C.A., Malik M.R., Elkholy A., Cauchemez S., van Kerkhove M.D. 'Worldwide reduction in MERS cases and deaths since 2016'. *Emerging Infectious Diseases*. 2019; 25(9): 1758–60. doi:10.3201/eid2509.190143

25. 'Prioritizing diseases for research and development in emergency contexts'. WHO. Accessed 20 August 2020. https://www.who.int/activities/prioritizing-diseases-for-research-and-development-in-emergency-contexts

26. 'We knew disease X was coming. It's here now. *New York Times*. Accessed 20 August 2020. https://www.nytimes.com/2020/02/27/opinion/coronavirus-pandemics.html

27. 'Blinking red: 25 missed pandemic warning signs'. *Genetic Engineering & Biotechnology News*. Accessed 22 November 2020. https://www.genengnews.com/a-lists/blinking-red-25-missed-pandemic-warning-signs/

28. 'Eli Lilly's antibody treatment gets emergency FDA approval'. *New York Times*. Accessed 10 November 2020. https://www.nytimes.com/2020/11/09/health/covid-antibody-treatment-eli-lilly.html

29. Cohen J. 'Champagne and questions greet first data showing that a COVID-19 vaccine works'. *Science*. Published online 9 November 2020. doi:10.1126/science.abf6414

## Chapter 2: Origins

1. Huang C., Wang Y., Li X., et al. 'Clinical features of patients infected with 2019 novel coronavirus in Wuhan, China'. *Lancet*. 2020; 395 (10223): 497–506. doi:10.1016/S0140-6736(20)30183-5

2. Zhu N., Zhang D., Wang W., et al. 'A novel coronavirus from patients with pneumonia in China, 2019'. *New England Journal of Medicine*. 2020; 382(8): 727–33. doi:10.1056/NEJMoa2001017

3. WHO. 'Pneumonia of unknown cause: China'. Accessed 20 August 2020. https://www.who.int/csr/don/05-january-2020-pneumonia-of-unkown-cause-china/en/

4. WHO. 'Novel Coronavirus: China'. Accessed 20 August 2020. https://www.who.int/csr/don/12-january-2020-novel-coronavirus-china/en/

5. Gorbalenya A.E., Baker S.C., Baric R.S., et al. 'The species severe acute respiratory syndrome-related coronavirus: classifying 2019-nCoV and naming it SARS-CoV-2'. *Nature Microbiology*. 2020; 5(4): 536–44. doi:10.1038/s41564-020-0695-z

6. Callaway E. 'The coronavirus is mutating: does it matter?' *Nature*. 2020; 585(7824): 174–77. doi:10.1038/d41586-020-02544-6

7. Chan J.F.W., Yuan S., Kok K.H., et al. 'A familial cluster of pneumonia associated with the 2019 novel coronavirus indicating person-to-person transmission: a study of a family cluster'. *Lancet*. 2020; 395(10223): 514–23. doi:10.1016/S0140-6736(20)30154-9

8. Chinazzi M., Davis J.T., Ajelli M., et al. 'The effect of travel restrictions on the spread of the 2019 novel coronavirus (COVID-19) outbreak'. *Science*. 2020; 368(6489): 395-400. doi:10.1126/science.aba9757

9. Zhang Y.Z., Holmes E.C. 'A genomic perspective on the origin and emergence of SARS-CoV-2'. *Cell*. 2020; 181(2): 223–27. doi:10.1016/j.cell.2020.03.035

10. Zhou P., Yang X.L., Wang X.G., et al. 'A pneumonia outbreak associated with a new coronavirus of probable bat origin'. *Nature*. 2020; 579(7798): 270–73. doi:10.1038/s41586-020-2012-7

11. Zhang T., Wu Q., Zhang Z. 'Probable pangolin origin of SARS-CoV-2 associated with the COVID-19 outbreak'. *Current Biology*. 2020; 30(7): 1346-1351.e2. doi:10.1016/j.cub.2020.03.022

12. Relman D.A. 'To stop the next pandemic, we need to unravel the origins of COVID-19'. *Proceedings of the National Academy of Sciences of the United States of America*. Published online 3 November 2020. doi:10.1073/pnas.2021133117

13. Boni M.F., Lemey P., Jiang X., et al. 'Evolutionary origins of the SARS-CoV-2 sarbecovirus lineage responsible for the COVID-19 pandemic'.

*Nature Microbiology.* Published online 28 July 2020: 1–10. doi:10.1038/s41564-020-0771-4

14. Wong A.C.P., Li X., Lau S.K.P., Woo P.C.Y. 'Global epidemiology of bat coronaviruses'. *Viruses.* 2019; 11(2). doi:10.3390/v11020174

15. Fan Y., Zhao K., Shi Z.L., Zhou P. 'Bat coronaviruses in China'. *Viruses.* 2019; 11(3). doi:10.3390/v11030210

16. Wang N., Li S.Y., Yang X. Lou, et al. 'Serological evidence of bat SARS-related coronavirus infection in humans, China'. *Virologica Sinica.* 2018; 33(1): 104–107. doi:10.1007/s12250-018-0012-7

17. Zhang Y.Z., Holmes E.C. 'A genomic perspective on the origin and emergence of SARS-CoV-2'. *Cell.* 2020; 181(2): 223–27. doi:10.1016/j.cell.2020.03.035

18. Wan Y., Shang J., Graham R., Baric R.S., Li F. 'Receptor recognition by the novel coronavirus from Wuhan: an analysis based on decade-long structural studies of SARS coronavirus'. *Journal of Virology.* 2020; 94(7): 127–47. doi:10.1128/jvi.00127-20

19. 'Seven more big cats test positive for coronavirus at Bronx Zoo'. Accessed 20 August 2020. *National Geographic.* https://www.nationalgeographic.com/animals/2020/04/tiger-coronavirus-covid19-positive-test-bronx-zoo/

20. Shi J., Wen Z., Zhong G., et al. 'Susceptibility of ferrets, cats, dogs, and other domesticated animals to SARS-coronavirus 2'. *Science.* 2020; 368 (6494): 1016–20. doi:10.1126/science.abb7015

21. 'SARS-CoV-2 in animals'. American Veterinary Medical Association. Accessed 20 August 2020. https://www.avma.org/resources-tools/animal-health-and-welfare/covid-19/sars-cov-2-animals-including-pets

22. Enserink M. 'Coronavirus rips through Dutch mink farms, triggering culls to prevent human infections'. *Science.* Published online 9 June 2020. doi:10.1126/science.abd2483

23. Oude Munnink B.B., Sikkema R.S., Nieuwenhuijse D.F., et al. 'Jumping back and forth: anthropozoonotic and zoonotic transmission of SARS-CoV-2 on mink farms'. *bioRxiv.* Published online 1 September 2020: 2020.09.01.277152. doi:10.1101/2020.09.01.277152

24. 'Denmark to kill up to 17 million minks after discovering mutated coronavirus'. *NPR.* Accessed 10 November 2020. https://www.npr.org/2020/11/05/931726205/denmark-to-kill-up-to-17-million-minks-after-discovering-mutated-coronavirus

25. Freuling C.M., Breithaupt A., Müller T., et al. 'Susceptibility of raccoon dogs for experimental SARS-CoV-2 Infection'. *Emerging Infectious Diseases.* 2020; 26(12). doi:10.3201/eid2612.203733

## Chapter 3: Coronavirus

1.  Abergel C., Legendre M., Claverie J.M. 'The rapidly expanding universe of giant viruses: Mimivirus, Pandoravirus, Pithovirus and Mollivirus'. *FEMS Microbiology Reviews*. 2015; 39(6): 779–96. doi:10.1093/femsre/fuv037

2.  Wasik B.R., Turner P.E. 'On the biological success of viruses'. *Annual Review of Microbiology*. 2013; 67(1): 519–41. doi:10.1146/annurev-micro-090110-102833

3.  Yin W., Mao C., Luan X., et al. 'Structural basis for inhibition of the RNA-dependent RNA polymerase from SARS-CoV-2 by remdesivir'. *Science* 2020; 368(6498): 1499–1504. doi:10.1126/science.abc1560

4.  Alberts B., Johnson A., Lewis J., Raff M., Roberts K., Walter P. 'Cell biology of infection'. *Molecular Biology of the Cell*. Published online 2002. Accessed 20 August 2020. https://www.ncbi.nlm.nih.gov/books/NBK26833/

5.  Gao Y., Yan L., Huang Y., et al. 'Structure of the RNA-dependent RNA polymerase from COVID-19 virus'. *Science*. 2020; 368(6492): 779–82. doi:10.1126/science.abb7498

6.  'What do we know about the novel coronavirus's 29 proteins?' Accessed 28 September 2020. https://cen.acs.org/biological-chemistry/infectious-disease/know-novel-coronaviruss-29-proteins/98/web/2020/04

7.  Finkel Y., Mizrahi O., Nachshon A., et al. 'The coding capacity of SARS-CoV-2'. *Nature*. Published online 9 September 2020: 1–9. doi:10.1038/s41586-020-2739-1

8.  Mahase E. 'Covid-19: First coronavirus was described in The BMJ in 1965'. *BMJ*. doi:10.1136/bmj.1.5448.1467

9.  Almeida J.D., Tyrrell D.A. 'The morphology of three previously uncharacterized human respiratory viruses that grow in organ culture'. *The Journal of General Virology*. 1967; 1(2):175–78. doi:10.1099/0022-1317-1-2-175

10. Enserink M. 'Calling all coronavirologists'. *Science*. 2003; 300(5618): 413–14. doi:10.1126/science.300.5618.413

11. Fehr A.R., Perlman S. 'Coronaviruses: An overview of their replication and pathogenesis'. In *Coronaviruses: Methods and Protocols*. Springer New York; 2015: 1–23. doi:10.1007/978-1-4939-2438-7_1

12. Menachery V.D., Yount B.L., Debbink K., et al. 'A SARS-like cluster of circulating bat coronaviruses shows potential for human emergence'. *Nature Medicine*. 2015; 21(12): 1508–13. doi:10.1038/nm.3985; Menachery V.D., Yount B.L., Debbink K., et al. 'SARS-like WIV1-CoV

poised for human emergence'. *Proceedings of the National Academy of Sciences of the United States of America.* 2016; 113(11): 3048–53. doi:10.1073/pnas.1517719113

## Chapter 4: Concepts

1. Hou Y.J., Chiba S., Halfmann P., et al. 'SARS-CoV-2 D614G variant exhibits efficient replication ex vivo and transmission in vivo'. *Science.* Published online 12 November 2020. doi:10.1126/science.abe8499
2. Grubaugh N.D., Hanage W.P., Rasmussen A.L. 'Making sense of mutation: What D614G means for the COVID-19 pandemic remains unclear'. *Cell.* Published online 3 July 2020. doi:10.1016/j. cell.2020.06.040
3. Kupferschmidt K. 'Mutant coronavirus in the United Kingdom sets off alarms but its importance remains unclear'. *Science.* Published online 19 December 2020. doi:10.1126/science.abg2626

## Chapter 5: Emergence

1. 'Intergovernmental science-policy platform on biodiversity and ecosystem services pandemics report: escaping the "era of pandemics" 2020'. Accessed 22 November 2020. https://www.ipbes. net/pandemics
2. Grandi N., Tramontano E. 'Human endogenous retroviruses are ancient acquired elements still shaping innate immune responses'. *Frontiers in Immunology.* 2018; 9(SEP): 2039. doi:10.3389/fimmu.2018.02039
3. Bos K.I., Harkins K.M., Herbig A., et al. 'Pre-Columbian mycobacterial genomes reveal seals as a source of New World human tuberculosis'. *Nature.* 2014; 514(7253): 494–97. doi:10.1038/nature13591
4. Faria N.R., do Socorro Da Silva Azevedo R., Kraemer M.U.G., et al. 'Zika virus in the Americas: Early epidemiological and genetic findings'. *Science.* 2016; 352(6283): 345–49. doi:10.1126/science.aaf5036
5. 'The natural history of Hardwar fair cholera outbreaks.' Accessed 15 August 2020. https://pubmed.ncbi.nlm.nih.gov/29002058/
6. Warren C.J., Sawyer S.L. 'How host genetics dictates successful viral zoonosis'. *PLoS Biology.* 2019; 17(4). doi:10.1371/journal.pbio.3000217
7. Kandeel A., Deming M., Kereem E.A., et al. Pandemic (H1N1) 2009 and Hajj pilgrims who received predeparture vaccination, Egypt'. *Emerging Infectious Diseases.* 2011; 17(7): 1266–68. doi:10.3201/ eid1707.101484

8.  WHO. 'Factors that contributed to undetected spread of the Ebola virus and impeded rapid containment'. Accessed 20 August 2020. https://www.who.int/csr/disease/ebola/one-year-report/factors/en/

9.  'Intergovernmental Science-Policy Platform on Biodiversity and Ecosystem Services Pandemics Report: Escaping the "Era of Pandemics" 2020'. Accessed 22 November 2020. https://www.ipbes.net/pandemics

10. 'Facial masking for Covid-19'. *New England Journal of Medicine*. Published online 23 October 2020. doi:10.1056/nejmc2030886

11. Warren C.J., Sawyer, S.L. How host genetics dictates successful viral zoonosis. *PLoS Biology*. 2019; 17(4). doi:10.1371/journal.pbio.3000217

12. Woolhouse M., Scott F., Hudson Z., Howey R., Chase-Topping M. 'Human viruses: Discovery and emergence'. *Philosophical Transactions of the Royal Society B: Biological Sciences*. 2012; 367(1604): 2864–71. doi:10.1098/rstb.2011.0354

13. Arunkumar G., Chandni R., Mourya D.T., et al. 'Outbreak investigation of Nipah virus disease in Kerala, India, 2018'. *Journal of Infectious Diseases*. 2019; 219(12): 1867–78. doi:10.1093/infdis/jiy612

## Chapter 6: Infection

1.  Lan J., Ge J., Yu J., et al. 'Structure of the SARS-CoV-2 spike receptor-binding domain bound to the ACE2 receptor'. *Nature*. 2020; 581 (7807): 215–20. doi:10.1038/s41586-020-2180-5; Wrapp D., Wang N., Corbett K.S., et al. 'Cryo-EM structure of the 2019-nCoV spike in the prefusion conformation'. *bioRxiv*. Published online 15 February 2020. doi:10.1101/2020.02.11.944462

2.  Bar-On Y.M., Flamholz A., Phillips R., Milo R. 'SARS-CoV-2 (Covid-19) by the numbers'. *eLife*. 2020; 9. doi:10.7554/eLife.57309

3.  Ke Z., Oton J., Qu K., et al. 'Structures and distributions of SARS-CoV-2 spike proteins on intact virions'. *Nature*. Published online 17 August 2020. doi:10.1038/s41586-020-2665-2

4.  Turoňová B., Sikora M., Schürmann C., et al. 'In situ structural analysis of SARS-CoV-2 spike reveals flexibility mediated by three hinges'. *Science*. Published online 18 August 2020. doi:10.1126/science.abd5223

5.  Wang Q., Zhang Y., Wu L., et al. 'Structural and functional basis of SARS-CoV-2 entry by using human ACE2'. *Cell*. 2020; 181(4): 894–904.e9. doi:10.1016/j.cell.2020.03.045; Yan R., Zhang Y., Li Y., Xia L., Guo Y., Zhou Q. 'Structural basis for the recognition of SARS-CoV-2 by full-length human ACE2'. *Science*. 2020; 367(6485): 1444–48. doi:10.1126/science.abb2762

6.  Cagno V. 'SARS-CoV-2 cellular tropism'. *Lancet Microbe.* 2020; 1(1): e2-e3. doi:10.1016/s2666-5247(20)30008-2

7.  Fosbøl E.L., Butt J.H., Østergaard L., et al. 'Association of angiotensin-converting ezyme inhibitor or angiotensin receptor blocker use with COVID-19 diagnosis and mortality'. *JAMA: Journal of the American Medical Association.* 2020; 324(2): 168–77. doi:10.1001/jama.2020.11301

8.  Matheson N.J., Lehner P.J. 'How does SARS-CoV-2 cause COVID-19?' *Science.* 2020; 369(6503).

9.  Hou Y.J., Okuda K., Edwards C.E., et al. 'SARS-CoV-2 reverse genetics reveals a variable infection gradient in the respiratory tract'. *Cell.* Published online 23 July 2020. doi:10.1016/j.cell.2020.05.042

10. Shang J., Wan Y., Luo C., et al. 'Cell entry mechanisms of SARS-CoV-2'. *Proceedings of the National Academy of Sciences of the United States of America.* 2020; 117(21). doi:10.1073/pnas.2003138117

11. Zhang L., Lin D., Sun X., et al. 'Crystal structure of SARS-CoV-2 main protease provides a basis for design of improved a-ketoamide inhibitors'. *Science.* 2020; 368(6489): 409–12. doi:10.1126/science.abb3405

12. Ghosh S., Dellibovi-Ragheb T.A., Kerviel A., et al. 'β-Coronaviruses use lysosomes for egress instead of the biosynthetic secretory pathway'. *Cell.* 2020. doi:10.1016/j.cell.2020.10.039

13. Cyranoski D. 'Profile of a killer: the complex biology powering the coronavirus pandemic'. *Nature.* 2020; 581(7806): 22–26. doi:10.1038/d41586-020-01315-7

14. Taber S.W., Pease C.M. 'Paramyxovirus: tissue tropism evolves slower than host specificity'. *Evolution.* 1990; 44(2): 435–38. doi:10.1111/j.1558-5646.1990.tb05210.x

15. Hoffmann M., Kleine-Weber H., Pöhlmann S. 'A multibasic cleavage site in the spike protein of SARS-CoV-2 is essential for infection of human lung cells'. *Molecular Cell.* 2020; 78(4): 779–84.e5. doi:10.1016/j.molcel.2020.04.022

16. Cantuti-Castelvetri L., Ojha R., Pedro L.D., et al. 'Neuropilin-1 facilitates SARS-CoV-2 cell entry and infectivity'. *Science.* Published online 20 October 2020: eabd2985. doi:10.1126/science.abd2985; Daly J.L., Simonetti B., Klein K., et al. 'Neuropilin-1 is a host factor for SARS-CoV-2 infection'. *Science.* Published online 20 October 2020: eabd3072. doi:10.1126/science.abd3072

17. Ibid.

18. Atyeo C., Fischinger S., Zohar T., et al. 'Distinct early serological signatures track with SARS-CoV-2 survival'. *Immunity.* 2020; 53(3). doi: 10.1016/j.immuni.2020.07.020

19. 'Eli Lilly's antibody treatment gets emergency FDA approval'. *New York Times*. Accessed 10 November 2020. https://www.nytimes.com/2020/11/09/health/covid-antibody-treatment-eli-lilly.html

20. 'FDA grants emergency authorization of antibody treatment given to Trump'. *New York Times*. Accessed 22 November 2020. https://www.nytimes.com/2020/11/21/health/regeneron-covid-antibodies-trump.html

21. Casadevall A., Pirofski L.A. 'The convalescent sera option for containing COVID-19'. *Journal of Clinical Investigation*. 2020; 130(4): 1545–48. doi:10.1172/JCI138003

22. Ibid.

23. Shen C., Wang Z., Zhao F., et al. 'Treatment of 5 critically ill patients with COVID-19 with convalescent plasma'. *JAMA: Journal of the American Medical Association*. 2020; 323(16): 1582–89. doi:10.1001/jama.2020.4783

24. Pathak E.B. 'Convalescent plasma is ineffective for COVID-19'. *BMJ (Clinical Research Ed.)*. 2020; 371: m4072. doi:10.1136/bmj.m4072

25. Chan K.K., Dorosky D., Sharma P., et al. 'Engineering human ACE2 to optimize binding to the spike protein of SARS coronavirus 2'. *Science*. Published online 4 August 2020: eabc0870. doi:10.1126/science.abc0870

26. Zoufaly A., Poglitsch M., Aberle J.H., et al. 'Human recombinant soluble ACE2 in severe COVID-19'. *Lancet Respiratory Medicine*. 2020; 8(11): 1154–58. doi:10.1016/S2213-2600(20)30418-5

27. Gardner M.R., Kattenhorn L.M., Kondur H.R., et al. 'AAV-expressed eCD4-Ig provides durable protection from multiple SHIV challenges'. *Nature*. 2015; 519(7541): 87–91. doi:10.1038/nature14264

28. Kiplin Guy R., DiPaola R.S., Romanelli F., Dutch R.E. 'Rapid repurposing of drugs for COVID-19'. *Science*. 2020; 368(6493): 829–30. doi:10.1126/science.abb9332

29. Zhang L, Lin D, Sun X, et al. 'Crystal structure of SARS-CoV-2 main protease provides a basis for design of improved a-ketoamide inhibitors'. *Science*. 2020; 368(6489):409–12. doi:10.1126/science.abb3405

## Chapter 7: Disease

1. Wiersinga W.J., Rhodes A., Cheng A.C., Peacock S.J., Prescott H.C. 'Pathophysiology, transmission, diagnosis, and treatment of coronavirus disease 2019 (COVID-19): a review'. *JAMA: Journal of the American Medical Association*. Published online 10 July 2020. doi:10.1001/jama.2020.12839

2.  Carfì A., Bernabei R., Landi F. 'Persistent symptoms in patients after acute COVID-19'. *JAMA: Journal of the American Medical Association.* 2020; 324(6): 603–05. doi:10.1001/jama.2020.12603

3.  Taquet M., Luciano S., Geddes J.R., Harrison P.J. 'Bidirectional associations between COVID-19 and psychiatric disorder: retrospective cohort studies of 62 354 COVID-19 cases in the USA'. *Lancet Psychiatry.* 2020. doi:10.1016/S2215-0366(20)30462-4

4.  Topol E.J. 'COVID-19 can affect the heart'. *Science.* Published online 23 September 2020: eabe2813. doi:10.1126/science.abe2813

5.  Ibid.

6.  Song E., Zhang C., Israelow B., et al. 'Neuroinvasive potential of SARS-CoV-2 revealed in a human brain organoid model'. *bioRxiv.* 2020; 6: 2020.06.25.169946. doi:10.1101/2020.06.25.169946

7.  Tay M.Z., Poh C.M., Rénia L., MacAry P.A., Ng L.F.P. 'The trinity of COVID-19: immunity, inflammation and intervention'. *Nature Reviews Immunology.* 2020; 20(6): 363–74. doi:10.1038/s41577-020-0311-8

8.  Stefely J.A., Christensen B.B., Gogakos T., et al. 'Marked factor V activity elevation in severe COVID-19 is associated with venous thromboembolism'. *American Journal of Hematology.* Published online 18 September 2020:ajh.25979. doi:10.1002/ajh.25979

9.  Ibid.

10. Cao W., Li T. 'COVID-19: towards understanding of pathogenesis'. *Cell Research.* 2020; 30(5): 367–69. doi:10.1038/s41422-020-0327-4

11. Moore J.B., June C.H. 'Cytokine release syndrome in severe COVID-19'. *Science.* 2020; 368(6490): 473–74. doi:10.1126/science. abb8925

12. Tan L., Wang Q., Zhang D., et al. 'Lymphopenia predicts disease severity of COVID-19: a descriptive and predictive study'. *Signal Transduction and Targeted Therapy.* 2020; 5(1): 1-3. doi:10.1038/ s41392-020-0148-4

13. Lucas C., Wong P., Klein J., et al. 'Longitudinal analyses reveal immunological misfiring in severe COVID-19'. *Nature.* 2020; 584: 463–69. doi:10.1038/s41586-020-2588-y

14. Laing A.G., Lorenc A., del Molino Del Barrio I., et al. 'A dynamic COVID-19 immune signature includes associations with poor prognosis'. *Nature Medicine.* Published online 17 August 2020: 1–13. doi:10.1038/s41591-020-1038-6

15. Laxminarayan R., Wahl B., Dudala S.R., et al. 'Epidemiology and transmission dynamics of COVID-19 in two Indian states'. *Science.* Published online 30 September 2020. doi:10.1126/science. abd7672

16. McDermott A. 'Inner Workings: Researchers race to develop in-home testing for COVID-19, a potential game changer'. *Proceedings of the National Academy of Sciences.* Published online 30 September 2020: 202019062. doi:10.1073/pnas.2019062117

17. Mina M.J., Parker R., Larremore D.B. 'Rethinking COVID-19 test sensitivity: a strategy for containment'. *New England Journal of Medicine.* Published online 30 September 2020: NEJMp2025631. doi:10.1056/ NEJMp2025631

18. 'Slovakia's mass coronavirus testing finds 57,500 new cases'. *Financial Times.* Accessed 10 November 2020. https://www.ft.com/ content/6d20007c-25ad-4d1a-b678-591acaa57df9

19. Ibid.

20. "FDA grants emergency authorization of antibody treatment given to Trump'. *New York Times.* Accessed 22 November 2020. https:// www.nytimes.com/2020/11/21/health/regeneron-covid-antibodies-trump.html

21. Hou T., Zeng W., Yang M., et al. 'Development and evaluation of a rapid CRISPR-based diagnostic for COVID-19'. Krammer F., ed. *PLoS Pathogens.* 2020; 16(8): e1008705. doi:10.1371/journal.ppat.1008705

22. 'Coronavirus: Tata Group to unveil India's first CRISPR test'. *The Hindu.* Accessed 25 September 2020. https://www.thehindu.com/ news/national/coronavirus-tata-group-to-unveil-indias-first-crispr-test/article32650334.ece

23. 'Feluda test kit to be made available in 8 metro cities'. *Hindustan Times.* Accessed 18 November 2020. https://www.hindustantimes.com/india-news/feluda-test-kit-to-be-made-available-in-8-metro-cities/story-sOAr6repyHYSWkkylPsGsK.html

24. Sethuraman N., Jeremiah S.S., Ryo A. 'Interpreting diagnostic tests for SARS-CoV-2'. *JAMA: Journal of the American Medical Association.* 2020; 323 (22): 2249–51. doi:10.1001/jama.2020.8259

25. Ibid.

## Chapter 8: Treatment

1. Mims C. *The War Within Us.* Elsevier; 2000. doi:10.1016/B978-0-12-498251-2.X5000-X

2. Couzin-Frankel J. 'From "brain fog" to heart damage, COVID-19's lingering problems alarm scientists'. *Science.* Published online 31 July 2020. doi:10.1126/science.abe1147

3. Kalil A.C. 'Treating COVID-19: off-label drug use compassionate use, and randomized clinical trials during pandemics'. *JAMA: Journal of the*

*American Medical Association.* 2020; 323(19): 1897–98. doi:10.1001/jama.2020.4742

4. 'Coronavirus disease 2019 (COVID-19) treatment guidelines'. Accessed 15 August 2020. https://www.covid19treatmentguidelines.nih.gov/

5. WHO Rapid Evidence Appraisal for COVID-19 Therapies (REACT) Working Group, Sterne J.A.C., Murthy S., et al. 'Association between administration of systemic corticosteroids and mortality among critically ill patients with COVID-19: a meta analysis'. *JAMA: Journal of the American Medical Association.* Published online 2 September 2020. doi: 10.1001/jama.2020.17023

6. FDA Approves First Treatment for COVID-19. FDA. Accessed 10 November 2020. https://www.fda.gov/news-events/press-announcements/fda-approves-first-treatment-covid-19

7. Dyer O. 'Covid-19: Remdesivir has little or no impact on survival, WHO trial shows'. *BMJ (Clinical Research Ed.).* 2020; 371: m4057. doi:10.1136/bmj.m4057

8. 'WHO rejects antiviral drug remdesivir as a COVID-19 treatment'. *New York Times.* Accessed 18 November 2020. https://www.nytimes.com/2020/11/19/health/Covid-WHO-remdesivir.html

9. Cai Q, Yang M., Liu D., et al. 'Experimental treatment with favipiravir for COVID-19: an open-label control study'. *Engineering.* Published online 18 March 2020. doi:10.1016/j.eng.2020.03.007

10. 'WHO rejects antiviral drug remdesivir as a COVID-19 treatment'. *New York Times.* Accessed 18 November 2020. https://www.nytimes.com/2020/11/19/health/Covid-WHO-remdesivir.html

11. RECOVERY Collaborative Group, Horby P., Lim W.S., et al. 'Dexamethasone in hospitalized patients with COVID-19: preliminary report'. *New England Journal of Medicine.* Published online 17 July 2020. doi:10.1056/NEJMoa2021436

12. 'Corticosteroids for COVID-19'. WHO. Accessed 4 September 2020. https://www.who.int/publications/i/item/WHO-2019-nCoV-Corticosteroids-2020.1

13. 'Association between administration of systemic corticosteroids and mortality among critically ill patients with COVID-19: a meta-analysis'. *JAMA: Journal of the American Medical Association.* Published online 2 September 2020. doi: 10.1001/jama.2020.17023

14. Cao B., Wang Y., Wen D., et al. 'A trial of lopinavir-ritonavir in adults hospitalized with severe covid-19'. *New England Journal of Medicine.* 2020; 382(19): 1787–99. doi:10.1056/NEJMoa2001282

15. Cohen M.S. 'Hydroxychloroquine for the prevention of COVID-19: searching for evidence'. *New England Journal of Medicine.* 2020;

383(6):585–86. doi:10.1056/NEJMe2020388; Geleris J., Sun Y., Platt J., et al. 'Observational study of hydroxychloroquine in hospitalized patients with COVID-19'. *New England Journal of Medicine.* 2020; 382(25): 2411–18. doi:10.1056/NEJMoa2012410; Boulware D.R., Pullen M.F., Bangdiwala A.S., et al. 'A randomized trial of hydroxychloroquine as postexposure prophylaxis for COVID-19'. *New England Journal of Medicine.* 2020; 383(6): 517–25. doi:10.1056/ NEJMoa2016638; Cavalcanti A.B., Zampieri F.G., Rosa R.G., et al. 'Hydroxychloroquine with or without azithromycin in mild-to-moderate COVID-19'. *New England Journal of Medicine.* Published online 23 July 2020. doi:10.1056/nejmoa2019014; Hernandez A.V., Roman Y.M., Pasupuleti V., Barboza J.J., White C.M. 'Hydroxychloroquine or chloroquine for treatment or prophylaxis of COVID-19: a living systematic review'. *Annals of Internal Medicine.* 2020; 173(4): 287–96. doi:10.7326/M20-2496; Abella B.S., Jolkovsky E.L., Biney B.T., et al. "Efficacy and safety of hydroxychloroquine vs placebo for pre-exposure SARS-CoV-2 prophylaxis among health care workers'. *JAMA Internal Medicine.* Published online 30 September 2020. doi:10.1001/ jamainternmed.2020.6319

16. Wang M., Cao R., Zhang L., et al. 'Remdesivir and chloroquine effectively inhibit the recently emerged novel coronavirus (2019-nCoV) in vitro'. *Cell Research.* 2020; 30(3): 269–71. doi:10.1038/s41422-020-0282-0

17. 'WHO discontinues hydroxychloroquine and lopinavir/ritonavir treatment arms for COVID-19'. WHO. Accessed 30 September 2020. https://www.who.int/news-room/detail/04-07-2020-who-discontinues-hydroxychloroquine-and-lopinavir-ritonavir-treatment-arms-for-covid-19

18. 'FDA cautions against use of hydroxychloroquine or chloroquine for COVID-19 outside of the hospital setting or a clinical trial due to risk of heart rhythm problems'. FDA. Accessed 30 September 2020. https:// www.fda.gov/drugs/drug-safety-and-availability/fda-cautions-against-use-hydroxychloroquine-or-chloroquine-covid-19-outside-hospital-setting-or

19. 'Revised advisory of the use of hydroxychloroquine (HCQ) as prophylaxis for SARS-CoV-2 infection (in supression of previous advisory dated 23rd March, 2020)'. MOHFW. Accessed 30 September 2020. https://www.mohfw.gov.in/pdf/AdvisoryontheuseofHydroxychloro quinasprophylaxisforSARSC

20. Zhang X.J., Qin J.J., Cheng X., et al. 'In-hospital use of statins is associated with a reduced risk of mortality among individuals with COVID-19'. *Cell Metabolism.* 2020; 32(2): 176–87.e4. doi:10.1016/j. cmet.2020.06.015

21. Caly L., Druce J.D., Catton M.G., Jans D.A., Wagstaff K.M. 'The FDA-approved drug ivermectin inhibits the replication of SARS-CoV-2 in vitro'. *Antiviral Research*. 2020; 178. doi:10.1016/j.antiviral.2020.104787

22. Gordon D.E., Jang G.M., Bouhaddou M., et al. 'A SARS-CoV-2 protein interaction map reveals targets for drug repurposing'. *Nature*. 2020; 583(7816): 459–68. doi:10.1038/s41586-020-2286-9

## Chapter 9: Immunity

1. Iwasaki A., Yang Y. 'The potential danger of suboptimal antibody responses in COVID-19'. *Nature Reviews Immunology*. 2020; 20(6): 339–41. doi:10.1038/s41577-020-0321-6

2. Lucas C., Wong P., Klein J., et al. 'Longitudinal analyses reveal immunological misfiring in severe COVID-19'. *Nature*. 2020; 584: 463–69. doi:10.1038/s41586-020-2588-y

3. Mudd P.A., Crawford J.C., Turner J.S., et al. 'Distinct inflammatory profiles distinguish COVID-19 from influenza with limited contributions from cytokine storm'. *Science Advances*. Published online 13 November 2020: eabe3024. doi:10.1126/sciadv.abe3024

4. Vabret N., Britton G.J., Gruber C., et al. 'Immunology of COVID-19: current state of the science'. *Immunity*. Published online 16 June 2020. doi:10.1016/j.immuni.2020.05.002

5. 'First Covid-19 reinfection documented in Hong Kong, researchers say'. *STAT News*. Accessed 24 August 2020. https://www.statnews.com/2020/08/24/first-covid-19-reinfection-documented-in-hong-kong-researchers-say/

6. Gupta V., Bhoyar R.C., Jain A., et al. 'Asymptomatic reinfection in two healthcare workers from India with genetically distinct SARS-CoV-2'. *Clinical Infectious Diseases*. Published online 2020. doi:10.1093/cid/ciaa1451

7. Wajnberg A., Amanat F., Firpo A., et al. 'Robust neutralizing antibodies to SARS-CoV-2 infection persist for months'. *Science*. Published online 28 October 2020: eabd7728. doi:10.1126/science.abd7728

8. Gudbjartsson D.F., Norddahl G.L., Melsted P., et al. 'Humoral immune response to SARS-CoV-2 in Iceland'. *New England Journal of Medicine*. 2020; 383(18): 1724–34. doi:10.1056/nejmoa2026116

9. Dan J.M., Mateus J., Kato Y., et al. 'Immunological memory to SARS-CoV-2 assessed for greater than six months after infection'. *bioRxiv*. Published online 18 November 2020: 2020.11.15.383323. doi:10.1101/2020.11.15.383323

10. le Bert N., Tan A.T., Kunasegaran K., et al. 'SARS-CoV-2-specific T cell immunity in cases of COVID-19 and SARS, and uninfected controls'. *Nature*. Published online 2020. doi:10.1038/s41586-020-2550-z

11. Hassan A.O., Kafai N.M., Dmitriev I.P., et al. 'A single-dose intranasal ChAd vaccine protects upper and lower respiratory tracts against SARS-CoV-2'. *Cell*. 1 October 2020. doi:10.1016/j.cell.2020.08.026

12. Addetia A., Crawford K.H., Dingens A., et al. 'Neutralizing antibodies correlate with protection from SARS-CoV-2 in humans during a fishery vessel outbreak with high attack rate'. *medRxiv*. Published online 14 August 2020: 2020.08.13.20173161. doi:10.1101/2020.08.13.20173161

## Chapter 10: Vaccine

1. Buss L.F., Prete, C.A., Abrahim, C.M.M., et al. 'Three-quarters attack rate of SARS-CoV-2 in the Brazilian Amazon during a largely unmitigated epidemic'. *Science*. Published online 8 December 2020. doi:10.1126/science.abe9728

2. FDA. 'Development and licensure of vaccines to prevent COVID-19: guidance for industry, 2020'. Accessed 21 August 2020. https://www. fda.gov/regulatory

3. Escobar L.E., Molina-Cruz A., Barillas-Mury C. 'BCG vaccine protection from severe coronavirus disease 2019 (COVID-19)'. *Proceedings of the National Academy of Sciences of the United States of America*. 2020; 117(30): 17720-26. doi:10.1073/pnas.2008410117

4. Netea M.G., Giamarellos-Bourboulis E.J., Domínguez-Andrés J., et al. 'Trained immunity: a tool for reducing susceptibility to and the severity of SARS-CoV-2 infection'. *Cell*. 2020; 181(5): 969–77. doi:10.1016/j. cell.2020.04.042

5. Lipsitch M., Dean N.E. 'Understanding COVID-19 vaccine efficacy'. *Science*. Published online 21 October 2020: eabe5938. doi:10.1126/ science.abe5938; Krammer F. 'SARS-CoV-2 vaccines in development'. *Nature*. Published online 23 September 2020: 1–16. doi:10.1038/ s41586-020-2798-3; 'Draft landscape of COVID-19 candidate vaccines'. WHO. Accessed 13 November 2020. https://www.who.int/ publications/m/item/draft-landscape-of-covid-19-candidate-vaccines

6. Wajnberg A., Mansour M., Leven E., et al. 'Humoral immune response and prolonged PCR positivity in a cohort of 1343 SARS-CoV 2 patients in the New York City region'. *medRxiv*. Published online 5 May 2020. doi:10.1101/2020.04.30.20085613

7.   Wajnberg A., Amanat F., Firpo A., et al. 'Robust neutralizing antibodies to SARS-CoV-2 infection persist for months'. *Science*. Published online 28 October 2020. doi:10.1126/science.abd7728

8.   Grifoni A., Weiskopf D., Ramirez S.I., et al. 'Targets of T Cell responses to SARS-CoV-2 coronavirus in humans with COVID-19 disease and unexposed individuals'. *Cell*. Published online 25 June 2020. doi:10.1016/j.cell.2020.05.015

9.   Lederer K., Castaño D., Atria D.G., et al. 'SARS-CoV-2 mRNA vaccines foster potent antigen-specific germinal center responses associated with neutralizing antibody generation'. *Immunity*. 2020; 53(6). doi:10.1016/j.immuni.2020.11.009

10.  '2020 Breakthrough of the Year.' *Science*. Accessed 22 December 2020. https://vis.sciencemag.org/breakthrough2020/

11.  'Why moderna and Pfizer vaccines have different cold storage requirements'. Shots. *Health News: NPR*. Accessed 17 November 2020. https://www.npr.org/sections/health-shots/2020/11/17/935563377/why-does-pfizers-covid-19-vaccine-need-to-be-kept-colder-than-antarctica; 'Covid-19 vaccine from Pfizer and BioNTech is strongly effective, data show'. *STAT News*. Accessed 9 November 2020. https://www.statnews.com/2020/11/09/covid-19-vaccine-from-pfizer-and-biontech-is-strongly-effective-early-data-from-large-trial-indicate/; 'New Pfizer results: coronavirus vaccine is safe and 95% effective'. *New York Times*. Accessed 17 November 2020. https://www.nytimes.com/2020/11/18/health/pfizer-covid-vaccine.html

12.  Ibid.

13.  Diamond M.S., Pierson T.C. 'The challenges of vaccine development against a new virus during a pandemic'. *Cell Host and Microbe*. 2020; 27(5): 699–703. doi:10.1016/j.chom.2020.04.021

14.  Gao Q., Bao L., Mao H., et al. 'Development of an inactivated vaccine candidate for SARS-CoV-2'. *Science*. 2020; 369(6499): 77–81. doi:10.1126/science.abc1932

15.  van Riel D., de Wit E. 'Next-generation vaccine platforms for COVID-19'. *Nature Materials*. 2020; 19(8): 810–12. doi:10.1038/s41563-020-0746-0

16.  'Bharat Biotech begins Covaxin Phase III trials'. *Indian Express*. Accessed 22 November 2020. https://indianexpress.com/article/india/bharat-biotech-begins-covaxin-phase-iii-trials-7055237/

17.  Wadman M. 'Will a small, long-shot U.S. company end up producing the best coronavirus vaccine?' *Science*. Published online 3 November 2020. doi:10.1126/science.abf5474

18. Lederer K., Castaño D., Atria D.G., et al. 'SARS-CoV-2 mRNA vaccines foster potent antigen-specific germinal center responses associated with neutralizing antibody generation'. *Immunity.* 2020; 53(6).

19. 'Why Moderna and Pfizer vaccines have different cold storage requirements'. *NPR.* Accessed 17 November 2020. https://www.npr.org/sections/health-shots/2020/11/17/935563377/why-does-pfizers-covid-19-vaccine-need-to-be-kept-colder-than-antarctica

20. 'What to Expect after Getting a COVID-19 Vaccine'. CDC. Accessed 22 December 2020. https://www.cdc.gov/coronavirus/2019-ncov/vaccines/expect/after.html

21. Hassan A.O., Kafai, N.M., Dmitriev, J.P., et al. 'A single-dose intranasal ChAd vaccine protects upper and lower respiratory tracts against SARS-CoV-2'. *Cell.* 2020. doi:10.1016/j.cell.2020.08.026

22. 'Coronavirus vaccine by AstraZeneca and Oxford up to 90 percent effective'. *Washington Post.* Accessed 22 November 2020. https://www.washingtonpost.com/world/astrazeneca-vaccine-effective-coronavirus/2020/11/23/fa2ad7b6-2d69-11eb-9dd6-2d0179981719_story.html

23. Anderson E.J., Campbell J.D., Creech C.B., et al. 'Warp speed for COVID-19 vaccines: why are children stuck in neutral?' *Clinical Infectious Diseases:* Published online 18 September 2020. doi:10.1093/cid/ciaa1425

24. Peeples L. 'Avoiding pitfalls in the pursuit of a COVID-19 vaccine'. *Proceedings of the National Academy of Sciences of the United States of America.* 2020; 117(15): 8218–21. doi:10.1073/pnas.2005456117

25. Garber K. 'Coronavirus vaccine developers wary of errant antibodies'. *Nature Biotechnology.* Published online 5 June 2020. doi:10.1038/d41587-020-00016-w

26. Bollyky T.J., Gostin L.O., Hamburg M.A. 'The equitable distribution of COVID-19 therapeutics and vaccines'. *JAMA: Journal of the American Medical Association.* 2020; 323(24): 2462–63. doi:10.1001/jama.2020.6641

27. 'World Health Organization announces distribution plan for COVID-19 vaccine'. ABC News. Accessed 22 November 2020. https://abcnews.go.com/Health/world-health-organization-announces-distribution-plan-covid-19/story?id=73031332

28. Yot Teerawattananon, Saudamini Vishwanath Dabak. 'COVID vaccination logistics: five steps to take now beyond vaccine safety, efficacy and procurement lie licensing and delivery—nations must get ready'. *Nature.* 2020; 587: 194–96. Accessed 13 November 2020. https://www.nature.com/articles/d41586-020-03134-2

## Chapter 11: Parallels

1. Kilbourne E.D. 'Influenza pandemics of the 20th century'. *Emerging Infectious Diseases.* 2006; 12(1): 9–14. doi:10.3201/eid1201.051254
2. Taubenberger J.K., Morens D.M. '1918 influenza: the mother of all pandemics'. *Emerging Infectious Diseases.* 2006; 12(1): 15–22. doi:10.3201/eid1201.050979
3. Chandra S., Kassens-Noor E. 'The evolution of pandemic influenza: Evidence from India, 1918-19'. *BMC Infectious Diseases.* 2014; 14(1). doi:10.1186/1471-2334-14-510
4. Mahapatra A. 'Swine flu pandemic: Mission accomplished?' *ACS Chemical Biology.* 2009; 4(7): 485–86. doi:10.1021/cb9001552
5. Isaacs D. 'Lessons from the swine flu: Pandemic, panic and/or pandemonium?' *Journal of Paediatrics and Child Health.* 2010; 46(11): 623–26. doi:10.1111/j.1440-1754.2010.01912.x
6. Ibid.
7. Shortridge K.F. 'The next pandemic influenza virus?' *Lancet.* 1995; 346(8984): 1210–12. doi:10.1016/S0140-6736(95)92906-1

## Chapter 12: Prevention

1. Prather K.A., Wang C.C., Schooley R.T. 'Reducing transmission of SARS-CoV-2'. *Science.* 2020; 368(6498): 1422–24. doi:10.1126/science.abc6197
2. 'Facial masking for COVID-19'. *New England Journal of Medicine.* Published online 23 October 2020. doi:10.1056/nejmc2030886
3. Hamner L., Dubbel P., Capron I., et al. 'High SARS-CoV-2 attack rate following exposure at a choir practice: Skagit County, Washington, March 2020'. *MMWR* 2020; 69(19): 606–10. doi:10.15585/mmwr.mm6919e6
4. Li Y.Y., Wang J.X., Chen X. 'Can a toilet promote virus transmission? From a fluid dynamics perspective'. *Physics of Fluids.* 2020; 32(6): 065107. doi:10.1063/5.0013318
5. Bogler A., Packman A., Furman A., et al. 'Rethinking wastewater risks and monitoring in light of the COVID-19 pandemic'. *Nature Sustainability.* Published online 19 August 2020: 1–10. doi:10.1038/s41893-020-00605-2
6. Chu D.K., Akl E.A., Duda S., et al. 'Physical distancing, face masks, and eye protection to prevent person-to-person transmission of SARS-CoV-2 and COVID-19: a systematic review and meta-analysis'.

*Lancet.* Published online 27 June 2020. doi:10.1016/S0140-6736(20)31142-9

7. Larochelle M.R. "'Is It Safe for Me to Go to Work?" risk stratification for workers during the COVID-19 pandemic'. *New England Journal of Medicine.* 2020; 383(5): e28. doi:10.1056/NEJMp2013413

8. Schröder I. 'COVID-19: a risk assessment prespective'. *ACS Chemical Health & Safety.* 2020; 27(3): 160–69. doi:10.1021/acs.chas.0c00035

9. Goldman E. 'Exaggerated risk of transmission of COVID-19 by fomites'. *Lancet Infectious Diseases.* 2020; 20(8): 892–93. doi:10.1016/S1473-3099(20)30561-2

10. Chang S., Pierson E., Koh, P.W., et al. 'Mobility network models of COVID-19 explain inequities and inform reopening'. *Nature.* Published online 10 November 2020. doi:10.1038/s41586-020-2923-3

11. 'Facial masking for COVID-19'. *New England Journal of Medicine.* Published online 23 October 2020. doi:10.1056/nejmc2030886

12. Konda A., Prakash A., Moss G.A., Schmoldt M., Grant G.D., Guha S. 'Aerosol filtration efficiency of common fabrics used in respiratory cloth masks'. *ACS Nano.* 2020; 14(5): 6339–47. doi:10.1021/acsnano.0c03252

13. US Surgeon General on Twitter: 'Seriously people STOP BUYING MASKS! They are NOT effective in preventing general public from catching #Coronavirus, but if healthcare providers can't get them to care for sick patients, it puts them and our communities at risk!' https://t.co/UxZRwxxKL9 / Twitter. Accessed 20 August 2020. https://twitter.com/Surgeon_General/status/1233725785283932160

14. 'Masks don't just filter the air, they keep people away'. *Washington Post.* Accessed 27 August 2020. https://www.washingtonpost.com/

15. Goldman E. 'Exaggerated risk of transmission of COVID-19 by fomites'. *The Lancet Infectious Diseases.* 2020; 20(8): 892–93. doi:10.1016/S1473-3099(20)30561-2

16. 'How we know disinfectants should kill the COVID-19 coronavirus'. *Chemical & Engineering News.* Accessed 20 August 2020. https://cen.acs.org/biological-chemistry/infectious-disease/How-we-know-disinfectants-should-kill-the-COVID-19-coronavirus/98/web/2020/03

17. 'Food safety and the coronavirus disease 2019 (COVID-19)'. FDA. Accessed 15 August 2020. https://www.fda.gov/food/food-safety-during-emergencies/food-safety-and-coronavirus-disease-2019-covid-19

18. 'We are over-cleaning in response to COVID-19'. *Washington Post.* Accessed 22 December 2020. https://www.washingtonpost.com/opinions/2020/12/11/covid-19-airborne-transmission-cleaning-surfaces/

19. van Doremalen N., Bushmaker T., Morris D.H., et al. 'Aerosol and surface stability of SARS-CoV-2 as compared with SARS-CoV-1'. *New England Journal of Medicine*. 2020; 382(16): 1564–67. doi:10.1056/NEJMc2004973

20. 'National Academies Rapid Expert Consultation on COVID-19 Pandemic'. National Academies Press; 2020. doi:10.17226/25753

21. Ibid.

22. Ibid.

23. Choi E.M., Chu D.K.W., Cheng P.K.C., et al. 'In-Flight Transmission of Severe Acute Respiratory Syndrome Coronavirus 2'. *Emerging Infectious Diseases*. 2020; 26(11). doi:10.3201/eid2611.203254

24. 'SARS-CoV-2: Transmission Routes and Environments, 22 October 2020'. GOV.UK. Accessed 18 November 2020. https://www.gov.uk/government/publications/sars-cov-2-transmission-routes-and-environments-22-october-2020

## Chapter 13: Spread

1. Bonita Beaglehole R.R. *Basic Epidemiology 2nd Edition*; World Health Organization, Geneva, 2006.

2. 'Asymptomatic spread of coronavirus "appears to be rare," WHO official says'. CNN. Accessed 20 August 2020. https://www.cnn.com/2020/06/08/health/coronavirus-asymptomatic-spread-who-bn/index.html

3. 'WHO comments breed confusion over asymptomatic spread of COVID-19'. *Scientist Magazine*. Accessed 20 August 2020. https://www.the-scientist.com/news-opinion/who-comments-breed-confusion-over-asymptomatic-spread-of-covid-19-67626

4. 'Situation report-41 total and new cases in last 24 hours'. World Health Organization. Accessed 20 August 2020. https://openwho.org/courses/severe-acute-respiratory-infection

5. Lavezzo E., Franchin E., Ciavarella C., et al. 'Suppression of a SARS-CoV-2 outbreak in the Italian municipality of Vò'. *Nature*. Published online 2020. doi:10.1038/s41586-020-2488-1

6. Pollán M., Pérez-Gómez B., Pastor-Barriuso R., et al. 'Prevalence of SARS-CoV-2 in Spain (ENE-COVID): A nationwide, population-based seroepidemiological study'. *Lancet*. 2020; 396(10250): 535. doi:10.1016/S0140-6736(20)31483-5

7. 'COVID-19 pandemic planning scenarios'. CDC. Accessed 15 August 2020. https://www.cdc.gov/coronavirus/2019-ncov/hcp/planning-scenarios.html

8.  Oran D.P., Topol E.J. 'Prevalence of asymptomatic SARS-CoV-2 infection'. *Annals of Internal Medicine*. Published online 3 June 2020. doi:10.7326/m20-3012

9.  '80% of cases could be asymptomatic'. ICMR. Accessed 15 August 2020. https://www.livemint.com/news/india/80-of-cases-could-be-asymptomatic-icmr-11587404077691.html

10. Byambasuren O., Cardona M., Bell Phd K., Ba J.C., Mclaws M-L., Glasziou P. 'Estimating the extent of asymptomatic COVID-19 and its potential for community transmission: systematic review and meta-analysis'. *Official Journal of the Association of Medical Microbiology and Infectious Disease Canada*. 2020; COVID-19: Accepted version. doi:10.3138/jammi-2020-0030

11. He X., Lau E.H.Y., Wu P., et al. 'Temporal dynamics in viral shedding and transmissibility of COVID-19'. *Nature Medicine*. 2020; 26(5): 672–75. doi:10.1038/s41591-020-0869-5

12. 'COVID-19 pandemic planning scenarios'. CDC. Accessed 15 August 2020. https://www.cdc.gov/coronavirus/2019-ncov/hcp/planning-scenarios.html

13. Ip D.K.M., Lau L.L.H., Leung N.H.L., et al. 'Viral shedding and transmission potential of asymptomatic and paucisymptomatic influenza virus infections in the community'. *Clinical Infectious Diseases*. 64(6): 736–42. doi:10.1093/cid/ciw841

14. Mateus J., Grifoni A., Tarke A., et al. 'Selective and cross-reactive SARS-CoV-2 T cell epitopes in unexposed humans'. *Science*. Published online 4 August 2020. doi:10.1126/science.abd3871

## Chapter 14: Curve

1.  Qualls N., Levitt A., Kanade N., et al. 'Community mitigation guidelines to prevent pandemic influenza: United States, 2017'. *MMWR Recommendations and Reports*. 2017; 66(1): 1–34. doi:10.15585/mmwr.rr6601a1

2.  'The shape of epidemics'. *Boston Review*. Accessed 26 August 2020. http://bostonreview.net/science-nature/david-s-jones-stefan-helmreich-shape-epidemics

3.  Markel H., Lipman H.B., Navarro J.A., et al. 'Nonpharmaceutical interventions implemented by US cities during the 1918-1919 influenza pandemic'. *Journal of the American Medical Association*. 2007; 298(6): 644–54. doi:10.1001/jama.298.6.644; Mills C.E., Robins J.M., Lipsitch M. 'Transmissibility of 1918 pandemic influenza'. *Nature*. 2004; 432

(7019): 904–06. doi:10.1038/nature03063; Hatchett R.J., Mecher C.E., Lipsitch M. 'Public health interventions and epidemic intensity during the 1918 influenza pandemic'. *Proceedings of the National Academy of Sciences of the United States of America.* 2007; 104(18): 7582–87. doi:10.1073/pnas.0610941104

4. Qualls N., Levitt A., Kanade N., et al. 'Community mitigation guidelines to prevent pandemic influenza: United States, 2017'. *MMWR Recommendations and Reports.* 2017; 66(1): 1–34. doi:10.15585/mmwr.rr6601a1

5. 'Remember the flu? Coronavirus sent it into hiding, but at a cost'. Reuters. Accessed 26 August 2020. https://www.reuters.com/article/us-health-coronavirus-flu/remember-the-flu-coronavirus-sent-it-into-hiding-but-at-a-cost-idUSKBN2221PG

6. CDC. *Principles of Epidemiology in Public Health Practice, Third Edition: An Introduction;* 2006.

7. 'Evaluating data types: a guide for decision makers using data to understand the extent and spread of COVID-19'. The National Academies Press. Accessed 20 August 2020. https://www.nap.edu/read/25826/chapter/1#7

## Chapter 15: Lethality

1. 'Covid-19 appears far more lethal than flu based on antibody test results'. *Washington Post.* Accessed 21 August 2020. https://www.washingtonpost.com/health/antibody-tests-support-whats-been-obvious-covid-19-is-much-more-lethal-than-flu/2020/04/28/2fc215d8-87f7-11ea-ac8a-fe9b8088e101_story.html

2. 'Global COVID-19 case fatality rates'. CEBM. Accessed 15 August 2020. https://www.cebm.net/covid-19/global-covid-19-case-fatality-rates/

3. 'COVID-19 pandemic planning scenarios'. CDC. Accessed 15 August 2020. https://www.cdc.gov/coronavirus/2019-ncov/hcp/planning-scenarios.html

4. Laxminarayan R., Wahl B., Dudala S.R., et al. 'Epidemiology and transmission dynamics of COVID-19 in two Indian states'. *Science.* Published online 30 September 2020. doi:10.1126/science.abd7672

5. 'Inside China's all-out war on the Coronavirus'. *New York Times.* Accessed 15 August 2020. https://www.nytimes.com/2020/03/04/health/coronavirus-china-aylward.html

6. Vijay R., Perlman S. 'Middle East respiratory syndrome and severe acute respiratory syndrome'. *Current Opinion in Virology.* 2016; 16: 70–76. doi:10.1016/j.coviro.2016.01.011

7.  Mateus J., Grifoni A., Tarke A., et al. 'Selective and cross-reactive SARS-CoV-2 T cell epitopes in unexposed humans'. *Science*. Published online 4 August 2020. doi:10.1126/science.abd3871

8.  Wiersinga W.J., Rhodes A., Cheng A.C., Peacock S.J., Prescott H.C. 'Pathophysiology, transmisson, diagnosis, and treatment of coronavirus disease 2019 (COVID-19): a review'. *JAMA: Journal of the American Medical Association*. Published online 10 July 2020. doi:10.1001/jama.2020.12839

9.  Davies N.G., Klepac P., Liu Y., Prem K., Jit M., Eggo R.M. 'Age-dependent effects in the transmission and control of COVID-19 epidemics'. *Nature Medicine*. 2020; 26(8): 1205–11. doi:10.1038/s41591-020-0962-9

10. 'Children and schools during the COVID-19 pandemic: do school closures help?' *Mexical Xpress*. Accessed 30 September 2020. https://medicalxpress.com/news/2020-09-children-schools-covid-pandemic-school.html

11. Wadman M. 'Why COVID-19 is more deadly in people with obesity—even if they're young'. *Science*. Published online 8 September 2020. doi:10.1126/science.abe7010

12. Zambrano L.D., Ellington S., Strid P., et al. 'Update: characteristics of symptomatic women of reproductive age with laboratory-confirmed SARS-CoV-2 infection by pregnancy status'. United States, January 22–October 3, 2020'. *MMWR Morbidity and Mortality Weekly Report*. 2020; 69(44): 1641–47. doi:10.15585/mmwr.mm6944e3

13. Galasso V., Pons V., Profeta P., Becher M., Brouard S., Foucault M. 'Gender differences in COVID-19 attitudes and behavior: panel evidence from eight countries'. *Proceedings of the National Academy of Sciences*. 2020; 117(44): 202012520. doi:10.1073/pnas.2012520117

14. Bunders M.J., Altfeld M. 'Implications of sex differences in immunity for SARS-CoV-2 pathogenesis and design of therapeutic interventions.' *Immunity*. 2020; 53(3). doi:10.1016/j.immuni.2020.08.003

15. Zeberg H., Pääbo S. 'The major genetic risk factor for severe COVID-19 is inherited from Neanderthals'. *Nature*. Published online 30 September 2020: 1–6. doi:10.1038/s41586-020-2818-3

16. Pairo-Castineira, E., Clohisey, S., Klaric, L. et al. 'Genetic mechanisms of critical illness in Covid-19'. *Nature*. Published online 11 December 2020. https://doi.org/10.1038/s41586-020-03065-y

## Chapter 16: Infectiousness

1.  'Angela Merkel draws on science background in Covid-19 explainer'. *Guardian*. Accessed 26 August 2020. https://www.theguardian.com/

world/2020/apr/16/angela-merkel-draws-on-science-background-in-covid-19-explainer-lockdown-exit

2.  Zhang B., Zhou H., Zhou F. 'Study on SARS-COV-2 transmission and the effects of control measures in China'. *medRxiv.* Published online 18 February 2020: 2020.02.16.20023770. doi:10.1101/2020.02.16.20023770

3.  Lloyd-Smith J.O., Schreiber S.J., Kopp P.E., Getz W.M. 'Superspreading and the effect of individual variation on disease emergence'. *Nature.* 2005; 438(7066): 355–59. doi:10.1038/nature04153

4.  Endo A., Abbott S., Kucharski A.J., Funk S. 'Estimating the overdispersion in COVID-19 transmission using outbreak sizes outside China'. *Wellcome Open Research.* 2020; 5: 67. doi:10.12688/wellcomeopenres.15842.3

5.  Laxminarayan R., Wahl B., Dudala S.R., et al. 'Epidemiology and transmission dynamics of COVID-19 in two Indian states'. *Science.* Published online 30 September 2020. doi:10.1126/science.abd7672

6.  Ibid.

7.  Kupferschmidt K. 'Why do some COVID-19 patients infect many others, whereas most don't spread the virus at all?' *Science.* Published online 19 May 2020. doi:10.1126/science.abc8931

8.  Wallace M., Hagan L., Curran K.G., et al. 'COVID-19 in correctional and detention facilities: United States, February–April 2020'. *MMWR Morbidity and Mortality Weekly Report.* 2020; 69(19): 587–90. doi:10.15585/mmwr.mm6919e1

9.  Moriyama M., Hugentobler W.J., Iwasaki A. 'Annual review of virology seasonality of respiratory viral infections'. *Annual Review of Virology.* 2020; 7. doi:10.1146/annurev-virology-012420-022445

10. 'Global report: lockdowns start to limit Covid-19 spread in Europe'. *Guardian.* Accessed 12 November 2020. https://www.theguardian.com/world/2020/nov/12/global-report-lockdowns-start-to-limit-covid-19-spread-in-europe

## Chapter 17: Measures

1.  Laxminarayan R., Wahl B., Dudala S.R., et al. 'Epidemiology and transmission dynamics of COVID-19 in two Indian states'. *Science.* Published online 30 September 2020. doi:10.1126/science.abd7672

2.  Anderson R.M., Heesterbeek H., Klinkenberg D., Hollingsworth T.D. 'How will country-based mitigation measures influence the course

of the COVID-19 epidemic?' *Lancet*. 2020; 395(10228): 931–34. doi:10.1016/S0140-6736(20)30567-5

3.  Markel H., Lipman H.B., Navarro, J.A., et al. 'Nonpharmaceutical interventions implemented by US cities during the 1918-1919 influenza pandemic'. *JAMA: Journal of the American Medical Association*. 2007; 298(6):644–54. doi:10.1001/jama.298.6.644. Mills CE, Robins JM, Lipsitch M. 'Transmissibility of 1918 pandemic influenza'. *Nature*. 2004; 432(7019): 904–06. doi:10.1038/nature03063. Hatchett R.J., Mecher, C.E., Lipsitch M. 'Public health interventions and epidemic intensity during the 1918 influenza pandemic'. *Proceedings of the National Academy of Sciences of the United States of America*. 2007; 104(18): 7582–87. doi:10.1073/pnas.0610941104

4.  Kissler S.M., Tedijanto C., Goldstein E., Grad Y.H., Lipsitch M. 'Projecting the transmission dynamics of SARS-CoV-2 through the postpandemic period'. *Science*. 2020; 368(6493): 860–68. doi:10.1126/science.abb5793

5.  Ferguson N.M., Laydon D., Nedjati-Gilani G., et al. 'Report 9: impact of non-pharmaceutical interventions (NPIs) to reduce COVID-19 mortality and healthcare demand'. doi:10.25561/77482

6.  Ibid.

7.  'India under COVID-19 lockdown'. *Lancet*. 2020; 395(10233): 1315. doi:10.1016/S0140-6736(20)30938-7

8.  'Global report: lockdowns start to limit COVID-19 spread in Europe'. *Guardian*. Accessed 12 November 2020. https://www.theguardian.com/world/2020/nov/12/global-report-lockdowns-start-to-limit-covid-19-spread-in-europe

9.  Kupferschmidt K. 'Mutant coronavirus in the United Kingdom sets off alarms but its importance remains unclear'. *Science*. Published online 19 December 2020. doi:10.1126/science.abg2626

10. Kupferschmidt K. 'Ending coronavirus lockdowns will be a dangerous process of trial and error'. *Science*. Published online 14 April 2020. doi:10.1126/science.abc2507

## Chapter 18: Effectiveness

1.  'Coronavirus success story: how Rwanda is curbing COVID-19 goats and soda'. *NPR*. Accessed 15 August 2020. https://www.npr.org/sections/goatsandsoda/2020/07/15/889802561/a-covid-19-success-story-in-rwanda-free-testing-robot-caregivers

2.  'South Korea's emergency exercise in December facilitated coronavirus testing, containment'. Reuters. Accessed 15 August 2020. https://www.

reuters.com/article/us-health-coronavirus-southkorea-drills/south-koreas-emergency-exercise-in-december-facilitated-coronavirus-testing-containment-idUSKBN21H0BQ

3.  Iwasaki A., Grubaugh N.D. 'Why does Japan have so few cases of COVID-19?' *EMBO Molecular Medicine*. 2020; 12(5). doi:10.15252/emmm.202012481

4.  Dehning J., Zierenberg J., Spitzner F.P., et al. 'Inferring change points in the COVID-19 spreading reveals the effectiveness of interventions'. *Science*. 2020; 369(6500). doi:10.1126/science.abb9789

5.  Islam N., Sharp S.J., Chowell G., et al. 'Physical distancing interventions and incidence of coronavirus disease 2019: Natural experiment in 149 countries'. *BMJ*. 2020; 370. doi:10.1136/bmj.m2743

6.  'India under COVID-19 lockdown'. *Lancet*. 2020; 395(10233): 1315. doi:10.1016/S0140-6736(20)30938-7

7.  Gt Walker P., Whittaker C., Watson O., et al. 'Report 12: the global impact of COVID-19 and strategies for mitigation and suppression'. MRC Centre for Global Infectious Disease Analysis. doi:10.25561/77735

8.  Gupta, M., Mohanta S.S., Rao, A., et al. 'Transmission dynamics of the COVID-19 epidemic in India and modelling optimal lockdown exit strategies'. *International Journal of Infectious Diseases*. Published online 3 December 2020. doi:10.1016/j.ijid.2020.11.206

9.  'India moves into 2nd place for COVID-19 cases: coronavirus live updates'. *NPR*. Accessed 30 September 2020. https://www.npr.org/sections/coronavirus-live-updates/2020/09/07/910401174/india-moves-into-2nd-place-for-covid-19-cases

10. 'New cases of COVID-19 in world: countries'. Johns Hopkins University Coronavirus Resource Center. Accessed 25 December 2020. https://coronavirus.jhu.edu/data/new-cases

11. 'India coronavirus: migrant workers stranded by lockdown walk hundreds of miles home'. *Washington Post*. Accessed 13 September 2020. https://www.washingtonpost.com/world/asia_pacific/india-coronavirus-lockdown-migrant-workers/2020/03/27/a62df166-6f7d-11ea-a156-0048b62cdb51_story.html

12. 'Coronavirus lockdown: Activists say over 300 deaths related to lockdown troubles'. *The Hindu*. Accessed 13 September 2020. https://www.thehindu.com/news/national/activists-say-over-300-deaths-related-to-lockdown-troubles/article31491525.ece

13. Laxminarayan R., Wahl B., Dudala S.R., et al. 'Epidemiology and transmission dynamics of COVID-19 in two Indian states'. *Science*. Published online 30 September 2020. doi:10.1126/science.abd7672

14. 'India posts worst GDP slump of major nations as virus spikes'. Bloomberg. Accessed 4 September 2020. https://www.bloomberg.com/news/articles/2020-08-31/india-s-economy-plunges-by-record-23-9-after-harsh-lockdown

15. 'India unveils "underwhelming" $10bn stimulus for pandemic-hit economy'. *Financial Times*. Accessed 18 November 2020. https://www.ft.com/content/c0d23498-e91f-4f58-bebb-4237ed2d5398

16. Lai S., Ruktanonchai N.W., Zhou L., et al. 'Effect of non-pharmaceutical interventions to contain COVID-19 in China'. *Nature*. Published online 2020. doi:10.1038/s41586-020-2293-x

17. Salje H., Tran Kiem C., Lefrancq N., et al. 'Estimating the burden of SARS-CoV-2 in France'. *Science*. 2020; 369(6500): 208–11. doi:10.1126/science.abc3517

18. Flaxman S., Mishra S., Gandy A., et al. 'Estimating the effects of non-pharmaceutical interventions on COVID-19 in Europe'. *Nature*. Published online 2020. doi:10.1038/s41586-020-2405-7

19. 'The way in which it was executed, India's lockdown itself became source of virus's spread'. *Indian Express*. Accessed 18 November 2020. https://indianexpress.com/article/opinion/columns/coronavirus-lockdown-india-covid-19-cases-deaths-6494930/

## Chapter 19: Endgame

1. Kissler S.M., Tedijanto C., Goldstein, E., Grad, Y.H., Lipsitch M. Projecting the transmission dynamics of SARS-CoV-2 through the postpandemic period. *Science*. 2020;368(6493):860–68. doi:10.1126/science.abb5793

2. Moore K.A., Lipsitch M., Barry J.M. 'COVID-19: The CIDRAP viewpoint part 1: the future of the COVID-19 pandemic: lessons learned from pandemic influenza'. 2020. Accessed 15 August 2020. www.cidrap.umn.edu.

3. 'Experts predicted COVID-19 would come in waves now they say it's a "forest fire"'. Accessed 15 August 2020. https://www.sciencealert.com/experts-predicted-covid-19-would-come-in-waves-now-they-say-it-s-a-forest-fire

4. Vijgen L., Keyaerts E., Moës E., et al. 'Complete genomic sequence of human coronavirus OC43: molecular clock analysis suggests a relatively recent zoonotic coronavirus transmission event'. *Journal of Virology*. 2005; 79(3): 1595–1604. doi:10.1128/jvi.79.3.1595-1604.2005

## Chapter 20: Impact

1. 'Two million Delmarva chickens euthanized as virus hobbles processing'. *Washington Post*. Accessed 20 August 2020. https://www.washingtonpost.com/local/two-million-delmarva-chickens-euthanized-as-virus-hobbles-processing/2020/04/24/82fc93a4-865d-11ea-878a-86477a724bdb_story.html
2. 'A monkey in India stole COVID-19 blood samples from a lab worker'. *Live Science*. Accessed 20 August 2020. https://www.livescience.com/monkey-steals-covid-19-blood-samples.html
3. Bhala N., Curry G., Martineau A.R., Agyemang C., Bhopal R. 'Sharpening the global focus on ethnicity and race in the time of COVID-19'. *The Lancet*. 2020; 395(10238): 1673–76. doi:10.1016/S0140-6736(20)31102-8
4. Yancy C.W. 'COVID-19 and African Americans'. *JAMA: Journal of the American Medical Association*. 2020; 323(19): 1891–92. doi:10.1001/jama.2020.6548
5. Dyal J.W., Grant M.P., Broadwater K., et al. 'COVID-19 Among Workers in Meat and Poultry Processing Facilities—19 States, April 2020'. *MMWR Morbidity and Mortality Weekly Report*. 2020; 69(18). doi:10.15585/mmwr.mm6918e3
6. 'Negative oil prices: what does oil below zero really mean?' Bloomberg. Accessed 13 September 2020. https://www.bloomberg.com/news/articles/2020-04-20/negative-prices-for-oil-here-s-what-that-means-quicktake; 'Rice prices surge to 7-year high as coronavirus sparks stockpiling'. Accessed 13 September 2020. https://www.cnbc.com/2020/04/08/rice-prices-surge-to-7-year-high-as-coronavirus-sparks-stockpiling.html
7. 'Which countries were (and weren't) ready for remote work?" Harvard Business Review. Accessed 26 August 2020. https://hbr.org/2020/04/which-countries-were-and-werent-ready-for-remote-work

## Chapter 21: Aftermath

1. *Intergovernmental Science-Policy Platform on Biodiversity and Ecosystem Services Pandemics Report: Escaping the 'Era of Pandemics'*. 2020. Accessed November 22, 2020. https://www.ipbes.net/pandemics
2. Baylis M. 'Potential impact of climate change on emerging vector-borne and other infections in the UK'. *Environmental Health: A Global Access Science Source*. 2017; 16(Suppl 1). doi:10.1186/s12940-017-0326-1

3.  Brownlie J., Peckham C., Waage J., et al. 'Foresight. Infectious diseases: Preparing for the future. Future Threats'. GOV.UK. 2006. Accessed 15 August 2020. www.dti.gov.uk

## Chapter 22: Future

1.  Lederberg J. 'Medical Science, infectious disease and the unity of humankind'. *JAMA: The Journal of the American Medical Association.* 1988; 260(5): 684–85. doi:10.1001/jama.1988.03410050104039
2.  'Early CDC test kits were delayed because of contamination issues, HHS report affirms. CNNPolitics. Accessed 15 August 2020. https://www.cnn.com/2020/06/20/politics/cdc-test-kits-contamination/index.html
3.  Doshi P. 'The elusive definition of pandemic influenza'. *Bulletin of the World Health Organization.* 2011; 89(7): 532–38. doi:10.2471/BLT.11.086173
4.  'How the coronavirus will change our lives forever—from music to politics to medicine'. *Washington Post.* Accessed 19 August 2020. https://www.washingtonpost.com/outlook/2020/03/20/what-will-have-changed-forever-after-coronavirus-abates/?arc404=true